D1284581

DOCTORED

A TRUE STORY

Sky Curtis

INANNA Publications and Education Inc.
Toronto, Canada

Canada Council   Conseil des Arts   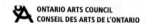 ONTARIO ARTS COUNCIL
for the Arts   du Canada   CONSEIL DES ARTS DE L'ONTARIO

We gratefully acknowledge the support of the Canada Council
for the Arts and the Ontario Arts Council for our publishing program.

We are also grateful for the support received
from an Anonymous Fund at The Calgary Foundation.   THE CALGARY FOUNDATION

Cover design: Val Fullard
Interior design: Luciana Ricciutelli

Library and Archives Canada Cataloguing in Publication

Curtis, Sky
        Doctored : a true story / by Sky Curtis.

ISBN 978-1-926708-18-8

        1. Curtis, Sky. 2. Curtis, Sky--Mental health. 3. Authors,
Canadian (English)--Ontario--Biography. 4. Sexually abused patients--
Ontario-- Biography. 5. Prejudices--Ontario. I. Title.

PS8555.U787Z463 2010   C818'.5403   C2010-906095-4

Printed and bound in Canada

Inanna Publications and Education Inc.
210 Founders College, York University
4700 Keele Street, Toronto, Ontario, Canada M3J 1P3
Telephone: (416) 736-5356 Fax: (416) 736-5765
Email: inanna@yorku.ca Website: www.yorku.ca/inanna

To Wendy who saved my life,
and to Mary who helped me live it.

Author's note: *This is my story and all the people I write about are real people. I have changed the names of everyone except myself.*

PROLOGUE

KATHY JUST LOVED ROLLING down hills. Her skinny body thumped over mounds of grass, arms and legs randomly flailing as she tumbled towards the bottom. Earth and sky flashed around her as she hurtled around and down. Finally she stopped, just seconds before hitting the hard packed gravel of the baseball diamond. Giddy with dizziness, she lay on her back watching the clouds swirl crazily above her. *Do it again! Do it again!* she sang to herself as she turned over to get up.

Suddenly a black shoe cracked against her teeth. She didn't see it coming. Her head snapped back and Kathy crumpled into a pile of skin and bones. When she could finally raise her head she saw her older brother Samuel a few feet away, staring at her, his hands in his pockets. Other kids were happily running around the schoolyard.

Kathy had a salty, rusty taste in her mouth. Blood. "Who kicked me?"

"I dunno," he replied, slouching away.

She ran home, her chin sticky with dark red blood. She hated the taste and kept spitting bubbles as she whimpered and ran. Her front tooth was gone. Her mother peered into her mouth and told her it didn't matter because she would get a new one soon. Kathy awkwardly dragged a chair over to the sink and washed the blood off her face, watching it turn the water pink before circling down the drain. Kathy was five years old.

*

Kathy stood in the backyard under the maple tree, dipping a piece of rhubarb into a paper cone full of sugar. She crunched on the stalk and watched her mother's dress swish around her legs as she hung the washing on the clothesline.

Sam stood swinging a golf club, sun glinting off the metal as he, at the age of seven, practiced his swing in the backyard.

"Stand back Kathy, stand back," he told her.

She was standing in the shade under the maple tree, watching him from the side of the sandbox. "I *am* standing back." There was lots of room. The sun flashed on and off the club as he swung it back and forth.

He took three steps towards her and swung the club high over his shoulder. As he whipped it toward her head he muttered, "I told you to stand back."

She heard the club's metallic thunk inside her skull. Disbelief coursed through her. She ran to her mother on legs she couldn't feel and collapsed into her arms. Her mother snatched a tea towel off the line and Kathy watched the approaching blue and white checks disappear into tiny pinpoints of light.

"Look, she's awake, her eyelids are fluttering."

Through her eyelashes Kathy could see a white surgical mask and dark brown eyes. A doctor was bending over her. He straightened up and squirted a small drop of clear liquid out of a thin needle. She watched the sharp metal point approach the side of her face and darkness rolled up from the back of her head.

Next she heard voices mumbling in the distance. Like waves on a beach they rose and fell in a far off echo chamber. Kathy's parents and the doctor were huddled together, their words swimming up through the murky depths: ..."It wasn't his fault... Don't be too hard on the boy... She could have died... He didn't mean it... She could have been blinded... Who gave him the club? It wasn't his fault... She's lucky to be alive... An inch up it would have been her temple... He didn't mean to... She is so lucky."

Kathy's tongue probed around in her mouth and she felt a string of rhubarb caught in her teeth.

Her whole head throbbed. *He meant it,* she thought. *But Mommy and Daddy said it wasn't his fault, so it must be mine. I'm such a bad girl. I'll try harder to be a good girl from now on. Then my brother will love me. Then he won't hurt me.*

Guilt settled into the marrow of Kathy's bones.

She went to school with two black eyes and her head wrapped in gauze. The kids laughed, "Ha ha ha, you're a raccoon. Kathy Raccoon." She was so ashamed of herself. Kathy was six years old.

*

A lady wearing a tight blue skirt was talking to Kathy's mother in the living room. The lady had a clipboard. Kathy couldn't really hear what they were saying because she was sitting cross-legged in the corner, in front of a blaring TV. Isolated words floated over the cartoons: "Stomach pumped six times. Two serious head ... hospital." They were talking about her younger brother, Daniel.

Kathy turned her head from the TV and watched the lady in the blue skirt rifle through papers, find one, and then tick items off a list. Her lips were puckered tight. She turned toward Kathy's mother. More words, "...Children's Aid ... warning."

Sam raced into the room. He was wearing an Indian headdress, its red and yellow feathers flapping, and he was whooping at the top of his voice. Daniel chased him, firing a small, engraved metal cap gun, hollering just as loudly. They circled around the lady, their grubby hands leaving shiny smudges on her skirt as they used her as a maypole. From the launching pad of her stiff body they hurled themselves out the front door, hooting and shooting into the street.

The lady tensed, smoothed her skirt down and then snapped the clipboard shut. "I see your problem." With her lips pursed and heels clacking lightly on the floor, the lady hurried toward the door and left without a backwards glance.

Kathy turned her head back to the TV. It wasn't her mother's fault.

*

Kathy and Sam crouched under the dining room table, playing astronauts. The drop leaves were down, creating a perfect spaceship. Bands of light shone through the cracks onto her brother's face. They were flying to Mars.

"I'm hungry, Astronaut Kathy," he said. "See the food up there, floating in space, through the crack in the spaceship? Reach through there and get me some."

Of course she would get some food for her brother. As she poked her fingers through the crack he lifted the drop leaf. Her fingers were trapped. He raised the table flap higher and higher until sharp, jagged pain jolted up her arm and exploded somewhere behind her eyes. She screamed. Just as she was beginning to faint she saw the hem of her mother's skirt twirling around her legs.

"There. That's done," her mother said as she patted the makeshift cast of popsicle sticks and gauze. "Your finger will be just fine in a week."

"I think it's broken." Kathy replied as she looked at the dressing doubtfully.

"It'll be fine."

That night lying in bed Kathy could hear her mother and father talking. Words floated out of sentences up the stairs: "...No hospital... No x-rays... Report... She'll be fine... It's not serious... Just a game... Not his fault..."

So. It was *her* fault. She deserved to be hurt. Kathy's finger pounded as she fell asleep. She would try harder to be good. If she was good she wouldn't get hurt.

Kathy had just turned seven.

*

Kathy watched lightning snake across the sky through the glass of the storm door. She could feel the thunder booming in her scrawny chest and wondered what it would be like to swallow electricity. She adjusted her upside-down ashtray crown, patted her dishtowel-veil into place, and became the beautiful and brave princess of light. Kathy ran outside through the downpour and clamped her lips around the lightning rod that ran down the side of the house. She waited. Later, while she was sitting at the kitchen table, she didn't remember much about what had happened, except that her teeth sang and her toes curled.

Kathy was at home alone because her mother was in the hospital. Her brothers were at a neighbour's. This was the second time her mother had been in the hospital. Her head wasn't right. But she was coming home soon. Tampax was on the kitchen table by the salt. Kathy had learned that women bleed after shock treatments.

She played with the pipe cleaner stickman her mother had sent her. It had arrived a few weeks earlier, folded up in a white piece of paper, her mother's bright red lipstick kiss dead center. Kathy held the paper up to her lips and kissed it back. The fear of not having her mother caused an electrical charge to shimmer all over her skin. Lightning zapped across her memory and she checked between her legs for blood. Nothing. She was eight.

*

All Kathy could hear was her own wheezing. She couldn't get any air. Her cat purred, curled up against her in her bed. Her mother was panicking. "Her lips are turning blue. Where's the damn doctor? She needs a shot of adrenaline, *now.*"

After what seemed like an eternity, the doctor's footsteps pounded up the stairs. Kathy glimpsed a glistening needle. Finally breath filled her lungs.

She didn't die. She knew she wouldn't. She never did.

The doctor glared at Kathy's mother. "Why is the cat in her bedroom? I told you the last time I was here: she's allergic to cats. Give the cat away. And you're a nurse!"

He stormed downstairs. The front door slammed and Kathy's mother looked at her and shrugged.

"I know it's not your fault, Mommy," Kathy whispered. "It was me who didn't want to give Tippy away." Not only was Kathy a bad girl, she was stupid. She was nine.

*

Kathy's family moved to a new house in a rich part of Toronto. It was huge with a big backyard and a leafy tree out front.

One day after school, Sam whipped a baseball at her head. A dark curtain fell across her brain. Floating sparkles of light danced in front of her eyes as she staggered up the back porch stairs to tell her mother. She called and called as the world tilted, but her mother wasn't home.

In the following months, Kathy had a growth spurt and her brother, at age eleven, did not. So, for a brief moment in their lives she was bigger than he was. One afternoon, while he was watching TV, she walked right up to him and slugged him in the nose as hard as she could.

"Take THAT!" she yelled. Kathy watched in horror as blood splurted all over the floor. But he never hurt her again. She was ten.

*

The night throbbed around her as her ears strained to pinpoint the source of the screaming. Was it her? The sound ricocheted inside her skull, bouncing off dark images, leaving echoes of shapeless terror. As she woke up a wheeze rattled in her chest and her hands were searching frantically through the sheets, the smooth texture of cold cotton catching on her damp palms.

She felt a soft warm fold of cloth. What had been there? Her cat? It must have been her cat. Yes, that's what it was. She was wheezing. Tippy had just left the bed, gone downstairs and was now howling to be let out. That's all it was. No one was screaming. Were they? Were her parents fighting again? All they did these days was fight.

Kathy tiptoed on ghost legs to her bedroom door and listened hard. Something shattered the vacuum of silence. What was that? She shrank against the doorframe, fear licking her skin. Another wave of silence drowned the house. Panic was balled tight at the back of her throat as she listened so hard she could hear the refrigerator humming in the kitchen below.

Kathy jumped as an ambulance siren suddenly sliced through the frozen January night. Just as suddenly, it stopped. She could hear wheels grinding up her driveway. She dodged the strobes of the flashing red light as she quietly made her way to the window. The pulsing light stopped while she was hugging the wall.

Her foot brushed against something on the floor and she jerked it back, recoiling in fright. It was her pink underwear. She felt her body disappear into fear. Night after night her underwear ended up on her bedroom floor. Perhaps she'd just forgotten that she'd taken it off. A few nights ago, before she went to bed, she had written a note to herself on the back of a chocolate bar wrapper: "Underwear ON." She had underlined the "ON" three times, to emphasize the point. The next morning her underwear was off. It was always off, on the floor. She didn't know why, but she knew it had something to do with all this.

Kathy stood beside the window and looked down onto the street from behind the net curtains. Nothing moved. Everything on the street was quiet and icy still. She stared for so long at the rough brown bark on the tree in the front yard that every detail became permanently etched on her retina. It felt as if the tree was rooted inside her. She saw its stiff limbs stretching upwards, silhouetted against the cold blue moonlight.

Two men got into the ambulance and drove it away. Who had it come for? What had happened? Kathy's cat stood stock still across the street watching the house. Its tail stood straight up, motionless in the cold, still air. But why was Tippy way over there? A cloud of steam rising from the sewer rolled over the cat and floated like a phantom into the shadows. A winter wind skittered stray leaves across the pavement. Tippy twitched her tail in the moonlight and the net curtains brushed against Kathy's skin. They felt like spider webs, trapping her.

She lay down in her bed and felt icicles of fear slicing through her veins. Her throat hurt. Was she the one who had been screaming? She didn't know. She felt like she no longer existed; she had disappeared. As she shivered under the cold blankets she felt like she had vanished into the gray static of TV snow. Kathy fell asleep with the white noise of fear crackling and hissing in her ears. It was somehow comforting.

*

Kathy got up early for choir practice and left for school in her oxford shoes, knee-high socks, pleated tunic, and white blouse. She was ten and could make her own breakfast. She had made a sugar sandwich and savoured the granules as they crackled against her teeth. Her bare legs went numb as she pressed against the freezing wind but she didn't care. She was going to sing.

She had fun at school that day: during art, she painted white swans with long necks on a pond; during science she reflected light off a mirror; and during geography she spun the shiny globe, feeling the slippery bumps of mountains and valleys sliding under her fingertips. After school she trotted to the corner store in the twilight and spent her allowance on a Crispy Crunch and a shiny green notebook.

That night she sat at her French provincial desk with the book open in front of her and knew she had to write. She had to figure something out. She couldn't write about the TV snow: way too frightening. Clouds, on the other hand, were manageable. She picked up her clickity pen, opened the book, and wrote her very first poem.

Then she wrote "private" at least ten times on the front of her shiny green poem book and put it in the desk drawer. She didn't want anyone to know how bad she was. She was doing something at night. She didn't know what it was, but her underwear was always on the floor in the morning. She was profoundly ashamed of who she was. She should die because of what she was doing. She locked the desk drawer.

That year she wrote poem after poem in her schoolgirl handwriting with carefully rounded letters and precise commas. She wrote about how she could walk on cold snow and not freeze because she was already dead. She wrote about how the ghost moon saw nothing but her blackened soul. She wrote about how death could be around the next corner. Every night she locked the book in her desk drawer. She had a secret.

*

A woman named Lynn had been living on the third floor of their house for months, ever since she had been fired as a nurse from the same hospital where Kathy's mother worked. Kathy was so proud of her mother because she was the Head Nurse of the Intensive Care Unit and kept very sick people alive.

But Lynn had been caught stealing drugs and was now working at a veterinarian's. Little vials of clear liquid medicines rattled in the fridge door whenever it was opened. Kathy didn't know what was in the vials but the tinkling of the glass frightened her.

One day Kathy's cat disappeared. She called and called "Tippy" out the back door and hunted under every porch in the neighbourhood. Lynn said the cat was sick and had to be put down. Kathy knew Tippy wasn't sick and knew Lynn had killed her. Once Lynn had sneered, "You love that cat, don't you?" and Kathy knew something poisonous had filled the room. Her heart ached. It was her fault Tippy was dead. She should have taken better care of her cat.

Her mother called Lynn "Lynny-poo," and told Kathy that Lynny-poo would get her a new cat from the vet. Kathy didn't hold her breath.

The stairs to the third floor were beside Kathy's bedroom. Whenever she heard them creak in the middle of the night she was rescued by the white noise of TV snow hissing in her ears. It sounded like rushing water and she swam downstream into the safety of sleep. Her underwear was always on the floor in the morning. She still didn't know why. Kathy was eleven years old.

*

Kathy's parents separated and she and her brothers moved to a smaller house with her mother and Lynny-poo. They were all ashamed to be living in the poor part of the neighbourhood and her mother deteriorated. Every morning she asked Kathy to bring her pills; either one red and two white, or two red and one white, depending. Her mother's hands would tremble, rattling her coffee cup on its saucer. Kathy felt desperately helpless as she watched her mother plunge into a dark sea of despair. It was Kathy's fault that she couldn't help her. She didn't know how. And that was because she was stupid.

The new house had wool carpets and they got a dog. Kathy's asthma grew worse and she often woke up in the middle of the night unable to breathe. She would wheeze into the bathroom and gulp down yellow medicine that tasted like licorice and take small blue pills. Then she would stand outside her mother's bedroom door, her hand poised to knock, just in case she suddenly needed to wake her up to call the doctor for a shot of adrenaline.

One night, as she stood shivering outside her mother's door, waiting for the medicine to kick in and wheezing in her thin nightgown, she could hear the sound of fists smacking against flesh. She was ashamed to her core that she did nothing, that she scuttled back to her bedroom, wishing she could disappear. The next day her mother had purple bruises up and down her arms. Kathy couldn't look at them.

*

Kathy made new friends at school. She became one of four smart and sassy girls who were velcroed together from the time they were eleven until they were well on their way to university. Mary Calderone, Mary Grisham, Mary Svenborg, and Kathy MacKay sat beside each other in most classes, often met up after school, and chattered gaily on the way to each other's houses.

The girls would sit around dining-room tables, talking endlessly about sex, drugs, music, and eating everything in sight. Kathy was grateful for the food as her mother's cooking had become sporadic. They never went to Kathy's house, which, fortunately for her, was in a far corner of the neighbourhood.

Kathy's home life had become increasingly violent. Lynn hit her regularly, her knuckles often aimed at Kathy's newly rounded breasts. Kathy knew she had to do whatever she could to survive. She kept out of the house and got involved in everything— sports, clubs, theater, and school politics—so she would have reasons to stay late after school. She ran everywhere. Running felt good.

And Kathy was good at running. She trained three times a week at school and went to track meets all over the province of Ontario. Finally, in a spectacular race, she became the fastest twelve-year-old runner of the one hundred yard dash. After the race she searched through the clapping crowd for a familiar face with her chest heaving and her hands on her hips. Her heart fell when she saw that no one from her family had come. But she was ecstatic on her way home and skipped up her street with the incredible news on her lips. She stood in the front hall and announced proudly to no one, "I won!"

Lynn had just come home from riding her horse and was standing in the living room wearing her riding boots and jodhpurs. She walked towards Kathy sniggering, "What? On those legs?" She flicked at Kathy's bare knees with her riding crop.

That familiar, frightening look of pleasure floated across Lynn's pupils and Kathy's blood began to hiss in her ears. She could feel herself vanishing into nothing as Lynn's foot began to slowly move backwards. Her leg snapped forward, the steel toe of her riding boot cracking against the side of Kathy's right knee. She didn't feel it connect.

Agony flowed like molten steel burning over her skin. Kathy could taste the pain, salty and bitter at the back of her throat. She stared hard at Lynn, refusing to cry. She limped upstairs, knowing she had made Lynn kick her. Kathy told no one. She was so ashamed of herself.

Kathy didn't run another race.

That night, Kathy hobbled downstairs in her nightgown to say goodnight to her mother and Lynny-poo, who were drinking in the living room. They were always drinking in the living room. Kathy could hear ice cubes tinkling against glasses and could smell cigarette smoke wafting through the air. She stood at the bottom of the stairs and said, "Nighty-night."

Lynn walked towards her with that same glint of menace and pleasure dancing together in her eyes. Kathy's heart began to pound as Lynn cornered her in the hallway, out of sight of her mother. The foul stench of alcohol enveloped Kathy as Lynn lowered her voice and hissed, "If you're so fast, run away from this."

A narrow column of flame shot out from the butane lighter Lynn had hidden in the palm of her hand. Kathy ducked as it singed her long hair. Terror electrified her body and she hopped on her good left leg up the stairs as fast as she could, her body contorting as she gripped and tugged at the banister. Screams of fear circled in her stomach but froze in her throat. She couldn't frighten her mother. She felt the flames brush against the calves of her legs. Lynn was right behind her. The fire flared at the hem of her nightgown, finally caught the material, and smoke curled around her.

Her brother's bedroom door slammed hard as Kathy struggled up the stairs. She burst into her room, flung the door shut, and twisted the lock. Lynn banged on the door, yelling in frustration. A volt of panic powered through Kathy's body and gave her the strength to push her heavy bookshelf against the door; it would never open now. Lynn went back downstairs and Kathy flung off her nightgown and stomped on it. She could hear whimpering. Was it her? She deserved to be set on fire.

*

During this first year in their new house her mother's mental illness slowly consumed her until she no longer went shopping for food or cooked. By July she had totally given up on feeding her children. On good days there might be some cereal and milk in the house but Kathy and her bothers were hungry all the time. Kathy found some baby-sitting jobs and became expert at taking food so no one would notice—a tangerine with a thin sliver of cheese, a cracker, a slice of ham. Nonetheless, she slowly began to starve. She fainted frequently and couldn't wait to get away to camp in August. Her father had started sending her and her brothers out of the city to old established summer camps the year before. Kathy loved camp with a passion. There someone took care of her all the time and she was fed three meals a day.

On the first day of camp she had to pass the mandatory swim test so she could go canoeing. She plunged into the cold water and fainted after her third crawl stroke. The next thing she knew she was in a hospital getting her blood tested for leukemia. Two days later she was diagnosed with malnutrition and left the hospital with the camp nurse, armed with huge iron pills and a twice-daily needle of something. The nurse told her she was lucky she didn't die. But Kathy felt lucky for another reason: Children's Aid hadn't been called in and she wouldn't have to betray her mother who was doing the best she could.

She liked the other girls in her cabin, but often felt herself watching them as if they were from another planet. Late at night she listened as they joked about the details of their most embarrassing moments, like getting lettuce stuck on a tooth or forgetting the words to a Beatles' song. Kathy joined in from the sidelines, laughing when they did, wishing she had problems like theirs. But she knew in her heart of hearts that it was she, not them, who was different.

*

When Kathy returned home from camp there was more food in the house. Maybe the camp director *had* called Children's Aid. Kathy, at the age of twelve, had just started going out with her first boyfriend. Lynn and her mother made jokes about him being Italian, not British. Kathy didn't care. She only knew that this boy was very nice to her and had the softest brown eyes she had ever seen.

One day, while she was getting ready for one of their dates, Lynn walked out of the kitchen with a knife flashing in her hand. Kathy raced towards the stairs, fear pulsing in the back of her throat. Lynn chased after her and grabbed Kathy's frail wrist as she tried to take the stairs two at a time. Lynn twisted her around and pinned her against the banister. Kathy recoiled in revulsion as Lynn's foul breath washed over her face.

"You going to show him your titties? Let's see them."

Lynn's eyes shone with malicious glee as she grabbed a fistful of Kathy's pale blue sweater and started sawing through it with the serrated blade. The sharp point kept nicking Kathy's chest as Lynn sliced back and forth through the acrylic fibers. Kathy froze; one wrong move would send the knife plunging into her heart. As Lynn sliced, Kathy felt as if flames of fear were burning the skin off her bones while she watched the knife slice back and forth through the fabric. Lynn finally ripped the frayed edges apart. She laughed at the new young breasts, her voice guttural and smelling of stale cigarette smoke. The world went gray and Kathy panicked that she would faint. But fear was revving in her muscles and she twisted herself free, running up the stairs on legs that seemed to have vanished, leaving Lynn at the bottom.

Kathy slammed her bedroom door and again struggled to push the bookshelf against it. She collapsed on the bed, crying and holding the frazzled edges of her sweater tightly together, the pale skin on her thin shoulders showing through the knitted fibers. As the fear slowly ebbed out of Kathy's body, a wave of shame swept through her. She felt so disgusting.

*

Suddenly, the attacks stopped! Did her mother tell Lynn to back off? Perhaps Lynn had turned her venom onto Kathy's brothers. Daniel ended up in the hospital in an oxygen tent with purple bruises around his throat. Had Lynn strangled him? And Sam mostly hid in the boys' bedroom. Kathy didn't know what was going on because she lived in a totally different world than her brothers. The dog was found poisoned under Kathy's bedroom window. She was no fool, she stayed out of the house as much as she could.

*

When Kathy was at camp she felt as if she were in heaven. Two full months away from her house! She had food. She had fun. She had love. She achieved in all the activities and was certain the camp director loved her more than anyone else.

After thinking long and hard, Kathy decided to let her camp counsellor read some of her poems. Two days later, Kathy stood at the bottom of the stairs to her counsellor's cabin, gripping the wire bound scrapbook she wrote in. Kathy could feel the wire cutting into her palm as she waited for the counsellor to say something.

"You are a writer," the counsellor proclaimed.

"I am?"

"Yes, you are a writer."

Kathy nodded as she digested the information. "Hmm," she said as she looked at her counsellor, "that explains a lot."

"What do you mean?"

Kathy grinned and held up her scrapbook. "I write."

Camp saved Kathy's life.

On the way home from a canoe trip in Algonquin Park, Kathy was told by her counsellor that she wouldn't be returning to her mother's house. That she and her brothers were going to live with her father. That he was hiring a cook. That the house was huge. No one told Kathy why, but she knew her mother wouldn't give up her children willingly. What had happened?

She lay in the back of the camp truck, her eyes glued to the clouds flying by as the news crept under her skin. Her heart ached with the thought of abandoning her mother, leaving her alone with Lynny-poo. Helplessness and relief roiled together in her chest while her tears dried in the wind as the truck sped over bumpy roads. When she got back to camp she had to skip around the dining room for her stupid fourteenth birthday.

*

Kathy's first year in high school flew by. She got high marks in all her courses, met a new boyfriend, swam on the swim team, and played volleyball. She liked the family cook and finally gained some weight. She was happier, but haunted by worry for her mother. Kathy and her brothers saw their mother just once that year, in May, at the new apartment she had to move into because she couldn't afford to keep the house. There was no sign of Lynn being there when the three kids visited, but Kathy knew Lynn was still in her mother's life. Kathy saw the bruises on her mother's arms, just visible under her thin white blouse.

Kathy looked around the apartment and saw the old familiar furniture from the house, the pearl inlaid end tables and the couch with the brocaded peacocks. Everything seemed to be the same for her mother, even the cut crystal decanters full of alcohol. Kathy had never seen her mother look so sad. She had been drinking, not a lot, not falling over drunk, but Kathy could always tell; she could smell alcohol a mile away. Kathy went down the elevator with despair in her heart. The following year she didn't see her mother at all. Kathy was fifteen.

*

The next July she left for camp again, and in the middle of the month the camp director called her to her cabin. Kathy thought she was in trouble for kissing her boyfriend, who had followed her to camp and worked in the kitchen. When she sat down on the sticky vinyl couch the camp director said, "Your mother died last night."

Kathy watched a speck of dust float in the sunlight. A distant radio played thinly in another room. She remembered her last visit to her mother's apartment. The bruises. The alcohol. The pills in the bathroom. Oh yes, Kathy had checked. Kathy's numbness at the news was pierced by a frightening question. What had happened?

"How?" she asked, her mouth suddenly dry.

The camp director's face was silhouetted black against the bright window. Kathy couldn't make out her features. "We're not sure. Perhaps there was something wrong with her heart."

Kathy's bare legs squeaked on the sofa. Her head began to hiss at her. TV snow. The director leaned forward. "The funeral's tomorrow. Do you have a dress at your house?"

"Yes," Kathy paused. She wondered if the dress she wore to the semi-formal would be appropriate for her mother's funeral. "Sort of. It's black and white, checked. Is that okay?"

The camp director's dusky voice calmed Kathy's rising panic. "I'm sure it will be fine. Someone will drive you back to Toronto tomorrow. Your brother's are being driven down from their camp, too. Everything's taken care of. "

That night all the girls in her cabin sat around whispering in the dark. They knew Kathy's mother had died and were being extra kind to her, making her laugh. In the far off distance they heard the rumble of a thunderstorm. Soon the slow sigh of deep breathing replaced the murmurs as everyone in the cabin fell asleep, one by one. But not Kathy. She felt so dirty.

Kathy unzipped her sleeping bag ever so quietly, grabbed her soap and towel and slid out into the night. She picked her way in the dark over roots and rocks, lifting her feet high so she wouldn't stub her bare toes. When she reached the lakeshore she put her soap and towel down on a rock and took off her nightgown. She stood quietly, watching the lightning zigzag across the sky.

She held her hand up in front of her face and began to tick off her fingers. "Don't swim in a storm. Don't swim alone. Don't swim after dark. Don't wash in the lake. Don't dive into shallow water." Kathy had run out of fingers. She lowered her arms down to her sides and opened and shut her fists, her thin body periodically illuminated by the flashes of light. Then she pointed at the lake, "And don't let your mother die."

Kathy did a shallow dive into the water, her splash barely rippling the surface. A jagged fork of lightning sizzled straight into the lake. A crack of thunder echoed through the air. Then all was quiet. A few bubbles floated on the black, shiny surface where Kathy had gone in.

She came up a good twenty feet away, her deep intake of breath softly filling the night. Then she quietly giggled; she had broken five rules with just one dive. Talk about efficient! But more than this, she knew lightning had struck the lake while she was underwater: she had felt the electricity humming on her skin. It had jangled in her teeth. It had vibrated in her eyes. But she didn't die! Who made up these stupid rules anyway?

She rolled on her back and floated, looking up at the stars. "Fuck 'em all."

Throughout the funeral Kathy felt like she didn't exist, like she was watching a movie and every now and then she'd see herself on the screen. She saw herself eating a sandwich triangle or how she was jammed between adults. She saw herself standing with her two brothers and noticed that their freckles looked like splatters of brown paint against pale gray skin. She couldn't cry. Images flashed around her eyes as faces suddenly darted in front of her, like attacking birds. Lipstick lips contorted and kissed her cheek.

Her aunt put an arm across her shoulder, passed her a Kleenex and said, "It's okay to cry. You must be very sad."

Kathy turned her face away from the claustrophobic perfume and muttered into the Kleenex, "Shut up shut up shut up."

Everywhere people were murmuring about what had happened. Her grandmother sailed into her vision and whispered, "Don't believe everything you hear," and whooshed out of sight. What did she mean? How had her mother died?

Kathy didn't know where her brothers had disappeared to in the crowd, but she was picked up before the funeral was over and whisked back to camp by two camp secretaries who drank and smoked for the whole two-hour journey. They bantered with each other while Kathy sat stonily in the back seat trying not to breathe in their cigarette smoke and alcohol breath. They stopped at a gas station and Kathy went into the bathroom to change out of her dress into a T-shirt and shorts. She balled the dress up into a tight wad and threw it into the garbage pail. The shiny lid swung back and forth, and Kathy watched her face vanish and reappear in the brushed metal. She felt like throwing up.

That night back at camp she lay in her bed and listened to the sounds of six other girls breathing around her. She shut her eyes and saw birds swooping and fluttering. They were shiny black, with wings the colour of dark, oily water. She could hear their feet scratching in what felt like dry, dusty dirt on the floor of her brain.

Kathy had birds in her head.

The next day she sat alone on a hill under a tree and looked around her. She looked and looked and looked at the forest, the road, the trees, the lake in the distance. She looked for what seemed to be hours. She knew she should cry, but she didn't. She knew she should be sad, but she wasn't. She wasn't anything.

Then she couldn't look any more and shut her eyes. She leaned against the tree with her lids squeezed shut and tried to imagine being part of it with roots reaching deep into the ground and branches lifting up towards the sky. When she opened her eyes she was terrified by everything she saw, so she would shut them again quickly.

In one of her glimpses she saw the camp's riding ring, dusty and waiting for the next group of campers. She quickly shut her eyes. Lynn's riding crop floated across her mind. Kathy's hand reached for the root jutting out of the earth beside her and she rubbed the bark.

That night in bed Kathy saw the birds again when she shut her eyes. And the next day she could hear them fluttering inside her skull, their wings brushing against her fear. She didn't let anyone know about the birds.

Three days later Kathy set out with five other girls and three guides on a two-week long canoe trip through northern Ontario. As she paddled through lake after lake she could feel her arms and back getting stronger. She felt the sun's goodness seep into her bones. Every stroke of her paddle took her further away from her mother's death.

One night, as she quietly lay on the ground by the campfire looking up at the stars, Kathy believed she could feel the heart of the earth gently beating as she lay on its soft skin. She felt her soul seeping down into the granules of dirt and floating up into the stars above. She felt that the land, the fire, the sky, the lake, and everything that existed, was entering into her whole being. She understood that there was an endless, good life force that ebbed and flowed through all things on earth, including her. She had found her god that night, under the stars, and she felt completely and deeply loved by this spirit of the earth. As she lay on the ground with her arms outstretched she received this love and felt a profound inner peace. She hugged herself and felt as if the universe was wrapped around her like a comforter. Then she whispered, "God is in nature."

On the way back to camp from the northern bush she once again lay in the back of the camp truck, looking up at the sky. The rhythm of the highway was jostling her into sleep and the memory of her last supper at her old house with her mother, grandmother, and brothers drifted through her mind. Lynn hadn't been there because Kathy's grandmother wasn't to know about Lynny-poo.

Kathy's mother and grandmother had sat at each end of the polished mahogany table, periodically checking on the manners of the three children. They talked above the children's heads, as if they couldn't hear. They were all eating spicy lamb curry. It was only slightly burnt; Kathy's mother had done her best to pull together a meal. Dainty slices of cucumber and banana waited on fine china side plates to soothe everyone's fiery mouths. Sterling silverware glistened in the glow from the long white tapered candles in the curling candelabra.

Kathy savoured the juicy curry while tuning in and out of the conversation. Her mother was talking about all the problems of being a single parent raising three kids alone. Her grandmother steered the conversation to the salvation of religion. Kathy's grandmother was very Church of England and believed that faith in the Christian God would solve everything. Her mother's laments were interrupted and dismissed by her grandmother's imperious English accent. "Now dear, if you just put your hand in the hand of God, all will be well," she chided.

Kathy jerked her head up. Then she whipped it back and forth from her mother to her grandmother. She wanted to watch what would happen next. Something would. Something really big. Her mother was an atheist, for Christ's sake.

Her mother's linen napkin rustled in the silence as she dabbed at her soft lips. To Kathy she was the most beautiful woman on earth. Her golden red hair shone softly like a setting sun in the candlelight. Her smile was so pretty, but the gaze from her metallic gray eyes pierced like a steel sword through the air across the table at her grandmother. The room had gone so still even the flames in the candles weren't moving.

And then a word shot out of her mother's mouth like the blast from a gun. "Balls."

Kathy's eyes went as wide as saucers. Her brothers snickered.

"Brown. Wrinkly. Hairy. Balls." Like buckshot, the words banged across the table.

The candles sputtered. So did her grandmother.

Kathy snapped her head down. Silent laughter burst in her chest, making her giddy and weak with delight. She loved her mother.

It was such a great memory. The corrugated metal of the truck dug into Kathy's back as the wheels whirred under her. Contentedly weak with exhaustion from the gruelling trip, the night swirled deliciously around her. She lay in a heap of sleeping girls, all bone weary from weeks in the bush. Almost sixteen years old, Kathy knew three things. She knew who she was: she was a writer. She knew what she believed: god was in nature. And she knew that she had spirit, just like her mother.

Kathy whispered into the wind, "Balls." What a great word.

*

Mary, one of Kathy's oldest friends, sat across from her in grade twelve history. The two of them were counting how many times their teacher cleared her throat. So far they had counted ninety-seven times. She had a throat problem, that's for sure. Mary clicked her tongue to get Kathy's attention and, once she had it, slowly lifted her hand to her nose and sniffed it. Then she mouthed the word "carbon." She tilted her head towards the athletic hunk in the third aisle over. Kathy and her three best friends had discovered that giving a guy a hand job made their palms smell like pencil lead.

Kathy was incredulous. Not the linebacker on the football team! They didn't go for the jocks. She mouthed back, her face screwed up in disbelief, "You did?"

Mary shrugged and offered her hand across the aisle for Kathy to smell as proof. Kathy pulled away and grimaced, "Gross."

The teacher cleared her throat extra loudly, her blue eyes fixed on the two girls. But what could she say? They got the highest marks in the class. Kathy looked down at her desk, crossed out the ninety-seven and recorded a big ninety-eight. She was seventeen.

*

Formaldehyde stung the inside of her nostrils as Kathy and Mary

Grisham bent over a dead rat. They had to dissect an animal for biology class. Its four little pink paws stuck straight into the air.

Kathy whispered to Mary, "It's good to get your feet up."

They collapsed into a fit of laughter. The teacher frowned. Kathy, knowing she was immune to a lecture with her ninety percent average, rolled her eyes.

He was not impressed and gave Kathy a warning look.

She bent her head intently over her rat and followed the diagrams precisely. To her it was so interesting, all the little organs and brain. She focused with all her concentration on being exact; the dissection was worth thirty percent of their final term mark. Kathy looked up when she heard Mary gag.

"Breathe through your mouth, Mare," she advised. "Then you won't smell it."

Kathy looked back down, and carefully cut a thin line down the middle of her animal. Suddenly her hand slipped, the surgical knife slid across the belly of the rat, and its white fur flapped apart.

"Shit. Just shit. I cut my penis off."

Her words hung in the silence of the classroom. And then everyone burst out laughing.

"Kathy MacKay" the teacher bellowed. "Go to the office. No swearing. And watch your pronouns."

Kathy gathered up her books, shrugged her shoulders while looking ruefully at the teacher and pretended to slink out of the classroom.

"It's not funny, Kathy." The teacher was furious.

"But sir, everybody's laughing." And they were.

She was eighteen.

*

Kathy was filling out her university application. She dug into her pocket for a quarter. She was going to flip a coin to choose her faculty. Kathy decided you had to be a bit of a bullshit artist to do well in the arts, so tails for arts, heads for sciences. Her whole future spun in the air and landed on the back of her hand. She looked under her palm at a majestic caribou. Tails. Kathy couldn't wait to leave home. But before she galloped off to Queen's University for a major in English, she went to camp.

There she taught waterskiing, swimming, and drama, all while taking care of seven rambunctious twelve-year-old girls. All the counsellors at the camp had to chose a nickname for themselves. Kathy couldn't think of one and finally the camp director christened her "Sky." Just like that, from then on almost everyone called her Sky. It was her new name for her new life away from home.

She was nineteen.

CHAPTER 1

WITH MY NEW NAME and happy hope in my heart, I thrived at university. I wrote for the school paper as a reviewer of Canadian literature and when my first ever published article came out, I actually held the newsprint to my nose and announced to my roommate, "This is the sweet smell of success." She looked at me askance. I was elected to be the Class Representative for at least one course a term. I wasn't sure if this was because I was popular or because no one else wanted to do the jobs that came with it, but I had a great time organizing speakers, dances, tutorials, social functions, fundraising, and staff reviews. Every weekend I went out with a bunch of kids and played Scrabble in the school pub while everyone placed bets on who would win. I gathered up my weekly take and used it to pay for my drinks and food. I didn't skip class, read what I had to, lost my virginity, and had lots of fun.

The next summer at camp I was promoted to run the drama program. Ella, a friend from the year before, poked her head into my cabin. "Aren't you going to bed?" she asked.

I slapped at a mosquito on my head. "I don't know how they expect me to be head of the camp's drama program when there are absolutely no plays for kids. This is the thirteenth adaptation I've written—Shaw this time."

"Yeah, well you're going to wreck your eyes, typing by flashlight, Sky," Ella replied. She looked skeptically at the flashlight I had rigged up, dangling from a rope and swinging in the breeze off the lake, its beam flickering across the old Corona typewriter. Ella was like that, kind and gentle. While Ella talked, I continued typing, my sweating fingers slipping off the damp keys and jamming in the bowels of the typewriter.

"Shit," I muttered. I tugged my finger out of the metal keys and lifted the bleeding cuticle up for Ella to see.

"Like my manicure?"

She rolled her eyes and laughed.

I was twenty.

*

I ran my fingers through my hair. It was only the beginning of May, but already it was hot. My friend Megan looked at me and asked, "So, where do you want to go?"

Megan and I had finally graduated from Queen's with Honours Degrees in English. Given how much fun I'd had, I thought it was a miracle I'd even passed and praised *Cole's Notes* daily. We were looking at a map of Europe spread out on Megan's bed.

"I'd like to go to the Norwegian Arctic when the sun never sets during the summer solstice, and to Wales to drink where Dylan Thomas drank, to sing in my chains like the sea." I replied, slurring the words and making Megan laugh.

Megan peered at the map intently. "I'd like to go here." Her finger was on the northernmost tip of Scotland.

And so it was that a few months later, Megan and I were leaning into a gale blowing in from the Atlantic as we gaped over the seaside cliff at the very north of Scotland. Down below were the carcasses of about fifty sheep, lying broken on rocks and being washed back and forth by the ocean's waves. The wind was so strong that I could feel my cheeks pressing against my teeth.

Megan looked at me and jerked her thumb to the herd of dead sheep at the base of the cliff. She bellowed over the howl of wind. "Sheep," she shouted. "They followed like sheep."

The bizarre yet horrific sight tumbled giddily in my chest, gathered steam and escaped in a series of laughing squeaks. Standing with my face tilted against the gale, barely able to move my mouth I squealed, "Don't make me laugh. I'm busy getting a face lift."

When we arrived in London, Megan and I stayed with one of Megan's family friends, Richard, a fun-loving, vibrant and charming man. We walked into his kitchen, and when he gave me a big hug I knew that this was the man I was going to marry. It was love at first sight. Over the next few days I discovered that we fit together perfectly. His whacky sense of humour was just like mine. He loved to play and so did I. His appreciation of nature was the same as mine. Plus I thought he was beautiful and couldn't keep my eyes off him. But would a long distance relationship work? It had to.

Because, at the age of twenty-three, I had found my one true love. And Megan and I had to go back to Canada.

Back in Toronto I felt like a mole tunneling underground when I took the subway to my first real job. I was working in an advertising agency and would pop out of the earth at King and Yonge and then take an elevator high in the sky. I was excited to be working, but my heart ached just to be outside, in nature. I felt I was working in a fishbowl, shuffling papers at a gray desk in a row of gray desks, the air a thick blue haze of drifting cigarette smoke. I couldn't get enough oxygen and felt like I was underwater.

I slumped at my metal desk and looked at a piece of paper that had been dropped into my 'In' box. It said "Affidavit" at the top. This was about the thirtieth piece of paper I'd received saying "Affidavit" at the top. I wasn't quite sure what the word meant or what to do with the papers so I kept stuffing them into the bottom right-hand drawer of my desk. After three months, the artistic director reviewed my performance.

"We all feel you've done very well here and would like you to take on the duties of media coordinator in addition to your current job of matching the Affidavits with the bills reflecting the radio time the client purchased."

Oh. So that's what they were for. How many Affidavits were in my drawer now? At least ten a day for about seventy days. I did the math. No wonder the small drawer could hardly shut.

I knew I was doomed in this job. There was no way I could possibly be a downtown business type of gal, so I stood up, shook the artistic director's hand, and said, "Thank you for your kind words. Thank you for all you've done. But I really don't belong here."

The director looked at me wide-eyed, mouth agape, while I hastily gathered up my purse. As my hand reached for the doorknob, I knew I had to tell the truth about the Affidavits. I turned around and said, "You might want to check my bottom right-hand drawer. Sorry. I'm really sorry." And then I bolted away. I never worked in an office again.

That night I wrote a long letter to Richard about what had happened.

I tried to make it sound funny, but no, it wasn't really. I knew he'd laugh about the Affidavits, but I had no job and rent to pay. With a sigh of resignation and a cup of tea, I sat at my desk. "Okay MacKay, now what?" I asked myself. I picked up my pen and wrote "now what now what now what" on a piece of paper. Then I sighed again. I was always writing. Mostly poems. A stack of shiny notebooks were piled on my desk.

"I'm a writer." I sighed with dismay. "That's what."

I took another sip of my tea and put it down a little more noisily than was warranted. "Great. A lifetime of being dead broke." I sighed again and shook my head.

"Fuck. Just fuck. *Fuck.*" Then I laughed. "Well Kathryn E., a.k.a. Sky, MacKay, for a writer you certainly have a way with words."

Resigned to my fate, I worked double shifts over the winter and spring as a waitress, slinging beer and flinging pizza. I saved every penny, bought an old car, and early in the fall drove to Nova Scotia to write by the sea. I landed in a small village called Robinson's Corner, found myself a house to rent, and set up a second-hand desk in front of a large sparkling ocean view; a perfect place for me to write poetry. After the hectic pace of downtown Toronto, I had some trouble adjusting to the slower pace of life in Robinson's Corner. I made up for the enforced calm by writing what I thought were hysterically funny letters to Richard daily, sending him amusing anecdotes about my new friends in Nova Scotia.

I was so pumped by my new adventure that I practically pranced to the local general store. I babbled to the store clerk, "What fabulous fresh produce you have here. Everything I could possibly want is in this store. That's so great; I live only half a mile away. Ten minutes walk. In a pretty little house with a fabulous view looking right across to Tancook Island. It's so great. Can I have a king size large Rothmans, please?"

The man behind the counter didn't look up and tossed me my smokes. I edged dejectedly out of the general store. What was *his* problem?

The next time I went into the store I only said, "Large Rothmans, please, king size."

The guy slid them across the counter and took my money. He was looking out the window and chewing on a toothpick.

Every day for the next six months I said the exact same thing when

I went into the store and he never said a word. Until one day.

I asked for my smokes. He gave me the change, looked at me slowly, breathed in, and asked, "Like it here?"

I looked him straight in the eye and sucked up a single word. "Yumph."

When I left the shop my head spun with glee. I'd been accepted into the community!

I leafed through the poems I'd written while gazing out to sea. These poems came from a mysterious place deep inside me and when I read them I really had no idea what exactly they meant. Nonetheless, I had enough material for a poetry reading. A few weeks later I read them to a decent crowd of my new friends who had gathered in a church hall in the nearby town of Chester. I was so proud of myself as I cut out the local paper's review and put it into a file. My career was beginning. I was a poet. My first review!

Every day I sent out copies of poems to various publishers. They'd boomerang back with rejection notices and I'd send them out again. I'd trudge through the fog to my mailbox and read pink slips until slowly, finally, some of them transformed into acceptances. A few began to be published in various literary magazines across the country. I had learned the trick of being a successful published writer: throw enough shit at the wall, some is bound to stick. I was almost twenty-four.

I typed and typed away on my electric typewriter in front of my large window looking out to the sea. As I typed I would say to myself, "These are the best days of my life. I am so lucky. I am *so* lucky. It is so beautiful here." The sun would sparkle on the ocean in the distance and I knew that god was certainly in nature here.

Over the next year I finished a novel, which was terrible, and filed it away. Then I worked for a small Atlantic news magazine and learned tons of production skills. I wrote a radio play about my long distance relationship with Richard and found a producer in Halifax who aired it on CBC Halifax Radio.

I was on my way. But I had to leave. The waitressing money was gone and I didn't see how I could earn any more in Robinson's Corner. I loved Nova Scotia so much; the landscape resonated inside my soul with a holiness that I cherished. With a heavy heart I packed up my old banger and headed back to Ontario where there was work. I was twenty-five years old, an adult.

When I arrived back in Toronto I immediately found an apartment near Ella's and another camp friend, Jordan. I had absolutely no money and still another old camp friend, Jane Wood, gave me the requisite first and last month's rent plus bought me a bed. That was so nice of her. Every month she sent me a hundred dollars until I had money from magazine articles coming in. She had utter faith in my ability as a writer. I connected up with two more camp friends who were now artists and started a syndicated children's column. I wrote videos, books, manuals, texts, whatever I could to make a buck. My career took off.

After a few years of writing letters to Richard and dashing across the ocean to see him, I was finally too frustrated by the distance; I had to get him to come to Canada. I begged and pleaded and finally, when I was twenty-eight, he arrived, his winter coat tucked over his arm. I took that as a good sign, given it was July! Financially it was hard. He wasn't allowed to work until he got resident status and painted houses for cash. But finally he could get a job and started at the bottom of the auto industry, selling cars. Time passed by incredibly fast as we got married, had children, bought a house, and worked diligently at our jobs.

By the time I was thirty-nine, I felt totally secure in my life.

CHAPTER 2

E LLA PANTED AS WE marched up a huge hill. "Now that you're forty, how are you feeling? A mid-life crisis?" she queried.

I could tell Ella anything. We were best friends, or BFs, as Ella called us. By now I had known her for almost two and half decades, ever since she'd laughed about my manicure at camp.

As I thought about her question, I could hear the cicadas humming in the forest.

I puffed as we hiked up and up under the hot summer sun. "I feel good about my life Ella." I told her. "I am happily married to the best man I've ever met. My kids are great. Emma and Margaret love their new school and are settling down. Jamie will soon be out of kindergarten and in full day school. I feel like June Cleaver, Ella. For the first time in my life even my finances are secure. My career is going gangbusters and Richard just had a great promotion."

"You've done well Sky," Ella said. "It's hard making a living as a writer and you've really worked at it. All those magazine articles, scripts, children's books, your syndicated column, the textbooks, the software designs. Man, have you ever worked hard."

"I know. But I'm worn out. Now that I can relax a bit I'm worried I might get sick."

"Naw, you're strong as an ox."

We climbed up the hill in silence until we were well past the brow and could breathe more easily. I was going over in my mind what I was going to work on next. A book on home-based science activities? A high school text on ancient civilizations? A grammar and composition program for schools? A science text?

Maybe Richard and I had enough money now that I could take a little time off from money-making projects and write fiction again. I hadn't written fiction since I had lived in Nova Scotia, a decade and a half earlier, and my heart soared with joy at the idea.

I broke the silence of the walk. "You know, I'm most excited about writing fiction, maybe a mystery book. I read them by the dozens, maybe I could write a good one. It would be so much fun to write fiction again."

"Well, you deserve it."

"Thanks Ella. But life's been pretty good to me lately. It was my childhood that was crappy."

"Yeah, that was pretty bad."

I sighed, "You don't know the half of it. In fact, neither do I."

"What do you mean, you don't know. You were there, weren't you?"

"Not really. I've blocked it out or something." I told Ella about the mysterious poems I'd written that had been published in my twenties. "One of them is about a cat, twitching its tail in the moonlight. Where does that come from? And another is about horses in a riding ring, of all things. I think they have to do with my childhood. I don't know what these poems mean. I don't know where they came from or even what they're about. My memory is weird like that. Every now and then I think about my mother and wonder how she died. It's been a haunting undercurrent in my life. I just wish I knew how she died. I tell people it was her heart, I mean, that's what I was told, but I don't know for sure. I keep getting this strange feeling that it was something sinister, but I don't know where that idea comes from. I get so scared sometimes, Ella, despite my 'perfect life' I always feel sort of jangled under my skin. It really bugs me, Ella. It has for years. Maybe she was murdered."

A seagull cawed in the distance as the word hung in the air.

The sun played across Ella's thoughtful face. "You can find out by writing to the Coroner's Office, Sky. They keep records."

The Coroner. Of course. I decided to do it.

When the response arrived in the mail, I nervously stuck my finger under the flap and sawed it open. The words of the Coroner's Report leapt around on the thick paper. I flipped through the pages, my heart racing. I read how my mother had been covered with bruises. Her left eye was swollen. A gash on her lip. Cuts on her legs. She had been drunk. Drugs were found in her body. There was a police report. *What on earth had happened?* The verdict was suicide. *Suicide?* What about the injuries? *She was still living with Lynny-poo. Could it have been murder?*

I felt terrified. What had lingered under my skin for years burst through and gripped me like a vise. My heart throbbed, my hands went numb, my head reeled, and I pitched forward. Would I fall right over? Throw up? My eyes were having trouble seeing through a sepia-coloured haze. I couldn't get enough air. My birds were back. I could hear fear beating its wings in my head. *Murdermurdermurder* whispered in my skull. And then I disappeared into TV snow, surprised at how familiar it felt.

Two weeks later the same thing happened in Canadian Tire, of all places. An almost complete collapse, with me holding on to my buggy for dear life so I wouldn't fall down. What was wrong with me? Did I have a brain tumour? Was there something wrong with my heart? Should I go to a doctor? I couldn't die, not yet.

There was Emma, Margaret, and Jamie to take care of and all those great ideas for projects. My mystery book. Richard. Perhaps an ear infection had made me lose my balance. I hated doctors but I knew I had to get checked out.

I was thumbing through my address book. What was my doctor's name again? I saw him so rarely. There it was, under "D" for "Doctor." Blackwood. Dr. Blackwood. The few times I'd seen Blackwood he'd seemed just okay. Not great. But doctors were so hard to find and I needed to see a doctor *now*. I pushed the number and got an appointment from a chirpy receptionist who identified herself as Lydia.

A week later my heart beat erratically as I sat in the waiting room. I was so nervous! Scared even. Doctors could tell you if you were going to live or die. Light reflected off the plastic nametag on the receptionist's fuzzy red acrylic sweater. So, this was Lydia.

I looked around the room. The place seemed so dingy. The carpet was stained, with coffee maybe, or perhaps tea, and the plastic on some of the chairs was ripped, the stuffing escaping in tufts. A hand-printed notice, "Leave Boots on the Mat" was taped to the wall, its yellowed edges curling. I located the source of a low staccato thrum; a fax machine was spewing out paper. A whiff of earth from the African violets on the window sill mingled with the sharp tang of rubbing alcohol. Cars on Bathurst Street were barely visible through the grubby windows.

Why were doctors always late? I had to pick up my kids.

And then my name was called.

Dr. Blackwood walked ahead of me out of the waiting room, turned right down a short hall and then took a quick left. His was the first door on the right. I stopped in the doorway while he walked straight ahead, turned around and sat behind his messy desk, facing me. He gestured for me to sit in one of the worn out mismatched chairs. One chair was torn and the other had a cushion with a brown stain on it. An examination table was on the right covered with ripped and crumpled paper. One edge of the venetian blinds dangled lower than the other, revealing another grimy window streaked with Toronto soot. An overhead fan light pulsed. Should I run? But I was desperate for help. *Please god, don't let me die.*

"How can I help you?" he inquired, his eyes penetrating.

More like "How could I help him?" I thought. I would hire him a cleaning lady, for starters. I had virtually raised myself as a child and my urge to parent this poor man who couldn't even keep his office clean surfaced from my heart to my throat. I gulped it back down. I flipped the stained cushion over and sat gingerly.

Dr. Blackwood looked endearing, sort of like a forty-year-old troll, his hair curling wildly around his ears. His electric blue eyes glittered, causing a hot jitter in my stomach. What did he remind me of? No, who? My heart started that pounding again. I was so dizzy. What did it all mean?

"I can't figure out why such strange things are happening to me and why I feel so scared. I know I'm exhausted; I've been working flat out for over ten years getting my career going, and now I think I might be collapsing and getting really sick. Last week I was in Canadian Tire pushing my cart down the electrical tools aisle when I could feel my heart knocking against my ribs. I had trouble getting enough air and kept trying to get more. Sort of gasping. My legs felt weak, like they were made of silly putty. You know that stuff? My mouth was stiff and my tongue felt like a piece of wood. I lost my balance and had to grip onto the handle of the cart so I wouldn't fall down. I felt so terrified that I would die."

He nodded, "And then what happened?"

He was writing in a file. Was he left-handed? Richard was. I loved Richard's hands. They were so capable and strong. I mentally turned my body around, trying to figure out if Dr. Blackwood was left-handed as well. I felt I was tilting inside my head and held on tight to the arms of the chair. The doctor looked at me askance.

"I, ah, went outside into the clear fall air—it was cool outside—and took a few deep breaths. I started to feel better after a few minutes."

Dr. Blackwood said, "I hate those stores. The fluorescent lights vibrate. Maybe that's what caused your problem. They rattled you, set you off." He made a large dismissive gesture with his hand, light glancing off his wedding ring.

I was quite certain my "problem" had nothing to do with lighting. I didn't understand why the doctor was being so dismissive. I kept probing. "Do I have a brain tumor? Or an ear infection? What's the matter with me? I'm worried I am very, very sick."

Dr. Blackwood told me to sit on the examining table and stood in front of me. The insect repellent smell of his aftershave made me wheeze. As he bent over my knee and gave it a minuscule tap with a tiny hammer, I could see the beginnings of a bald spot on the crown of his head.

While he was looking in my ears, I apprehensively asked him, "Do you see anything at all?"

He moved the waxy instrument around. "No, nothing."

I was giddy with relief. "Ah, so it's true, I really am an airhead," I joked.

A smile played about the corner of his mouth as he replied, "Well, you don't have a brain tumour."

So I wouldn't die. But what was wrong with me? I was late picking up the kids.

I was so exhausted that Richard and I had decided I needed a complete break from family duties, a holiday. So a few weeks later, I was relieved to be walking on a beach north of Halifax with a good Nova Scotian friend, Catherine Thorne. The icy Atlantic played at our shoes as we walked over the wet sand. Finally we found some quiet sunshine and began to eat the picnic she'd packed for us. Seagulls soared overhead, cawing for crumbs. My hands shook as I unwrapped the wax paper around the egg sandwiches. Catherine was a therapist, and she noticed these things. Looking at me questioningly, she asked how I was. As the sun beat down warmly on our backs, I described what had happened in Canadian Tire.

"That's an anxiety attack," she told me.

"Oh, that's it? That's all? What should I do?"

"Have you considered getting therapy? It might do you some good to meet with someone regularly, to talk about what's bothering you. Start with your family doctor."

"My doctor? Naw, he's pretty useless. And it's almost impossible to get a new doctor in Toronto. It'll go away."

Dr. Blackwood had no idea what was wrong with me. Fluorescent lights causing anxiety attacks? Where'd he get his education? But I knew I would have to do something, and soon.

Back in Toronto, I was driving on the Allen Expressway and my heart began to pound. *Oh, no.* Not while I was driving. I could hardly breathe. My arms and legs were disappearing into fire. My stomach churned and my mouth tingled. I was so terrified I could taste the fear. What was happening to my eyes? Would I have an accident? I crawled home on side streets, breathing deeply and waiting for my limbs to reappear. What if I died? What about Emma, Margaret, and Jamie? Richard? My work? I decided I couldn't drive on the highway anymore.

My life slowly shut down as my anxiety attacks increased. I lived in a state of terror. I couldn't take the subway. I couldn't take an elevator. I couldn't go up an escalator. I couldn't fly in an airplane. I couldn't go out on a balcony. I couldn't even clean the hamster. It wasn't long before there were a lot of things I could no longer do. Was I mentally ill like my mother? Oh god, please no.

I went to the grocery store with my teeth clenched, determined to buy vegetables. I needed to make sure the kids had three meals a day. I made lists of where I had to drive them. I watched them at all their events. I would not neglect my children. I would not be like my mother. But Catherine was right, I needed help. I needed therapy. Reluctantly, I decided to go back to Dr. Blackwood. In preparation, I wrote out the long list of activities that I now found impossible to perform. I counted them with dismay. Twenty-eight. I booked a morning appointment this time so I wouldn't be late again for my kids.

CHAPTER 3

GAIN I FOUND MYSELF sitting in the decrepit waiting room in front of the bouncy Lydia. Finally Dr. Blackwood appeared and called my name. I followed him into his gloomy office, sat down on the stained chair, and handed him my long list of problems saying, "Here is a list of twenty-eight things I can't do. A friend of mine told me I was suffering from anxiety."

Lights indeed.

He tilted back in his chair and took the sheet. "Ah. I was wondering what was going on with you." He adjusted his glasses as he peered at the list. "That's quite a list."

"Yes, my friend said I should get some help in dealing with this. She said I should talk to a therapist and that seeing my doctor would be a good place to start."

He looked at me over his glasses. "I could be your therapist," he offered. "I know what therapy is. I've been in therapy myself for the past two years. And, I'm accepting patients right now."

He'd been in therapy? Poor man. But should he be telling me this? How could he be helpful if he, too, were anxious? I felt so sorry for him, if he felt the way I did. The ceiling fan light vibrated above us. My hands were shaking again. "Your ceiling fan is slicing the light and making me frantic."

"Oh, sorry, I'll turn it off." He got out of his chair and glided past me, his hand outstretched towards the doorframe. There was a click behind me as he tried to turn off the fan, but both the light and the fan went off and the room was suddenly plunged into a shadowy darkness. Faint light filtered under the shut door and cloaked everything in a ghostly gloom.

I shuddered. I hated the dark. It was the first item on my list. Hadn't he just read the list? "Can't be in the dark." Fear consumed me. I could feel the shadowy air swoosh around me as he slid back into his chair.

He eased himself down and said in a low, soft voice, "There. No more vibrating light. We can start right now."

"I think if you pull that little chain dangling from the fan, just the fan will go off."

He looked at the chain and shrugged. Leaning forward in his chair, he said, "You can call me David."

There was something spooky about his eyes. I took a deep breath and tried to act normal. It was just anxiety. I wouldn't die. I was safe. I was in a doctor's office, for heaven's sake.

"Shouldn't I call you 'Doctor'? Or is it different if you're doing therapy on me?"

"Partners. We're partners." He paused meaningfully and I could see his eyes shining through the gray light.

I just knew I'd seen eyes like that before. Who's? Suddenly a violent feeling coursed through my veins. Was it fear? Or was I thrilled? It was such a big feeling, but I had no idea what it was. At the same time, everything felt sickly familiar.

Why couldn't I see straight? Murky images of his furniture swam around me. There was a part of me that wanted to run away from him, but I couldn't because it felt as if my legs had disappeared. And part of me was actually drawn towards him. It felt like there was a magnetic force coming off him, gripping me in its power. I quivered as the net curtains from my childhood bedroom floated across my memory. The memory made me shudder. Was I in danger or was I safe? Was I attracted to him or repelled? Why didn't I know? Maybe I was I simply trapped. He'd said "partners." A little voice whispered inside my head, "Said the spider to the fly."

But surely he wouldn't harm me. He was a *doctor* and he would help me get better. How bad could it get? I could hear my birds beating their wings hard inside my skull. The feeling, whatever it was, raced through me with an electrifying zap, charging everything I was made of with a revving energy.

I knew this revved feeling, even if I didn't know what it was called. I knew it like I knew my own skin. I clung to it like a life raft because it was familiar to me. I'd felt this before and I'd always been fine. I convinced myself I was okay. Something just below my ribs was trembling. I took a deep breath.

I felt like I had no choice. It was impossible to find a new doctor in

Toronto. I would try very hard to please him. I would do my best to be good. I wouldn't get hurt.

What on earth was I thinking? Nothing bad would happen. I was probably overreacting because of my anxiety. Dr. Blackwood seemed kind, considerate, but somehow sad and alone, somehow vulnerable. What had happened to him? Maybe he needed help too. My driving force to parent anyone who I thought needed taking care of overwhelmed me. I took another long slow breath while the room seemed to change shape. Bottom line was, I had to get better. It was somehow comforting to be feeling buzzed the way I was, to hear my birds. It was familiar. I'd be just fine.

"Why don't you come in next week and we'll start your therapy. Say, next Monday, that's just a few days away. Will you be okay until then?"

"Thanks, yes. I'll make an appointment on my way out."

Four days later I found myself sitting in front of Dr. Blackwood, no, *David*. He turned out the light and I could barely make out that he kept poking his glasses up his nose. Was it a nervous twitch? Maybe he was anxious because he really didn't know what he was doing. I remembered my conversation with Catherine on the beach. She was a good therapist. She knew what she was doing. Maybe I could help David along.

"This therapist friend of mine, Catherine, told me it's better to face the things that cause anxiety. She described a Buddhist meditation where the goal is to totally fill yourself with fear and then imagine you're breathing white light into the fear. This transforms the fear into a positive experience. It sort of 'flips' having anxiety about the event into loving the event. What do you think about all this, David?"

I felt awkward saying his name. He poked his glasses up his nose again. It looked like he was thinking. "Do you think it would work, David?"

"I'm willing to try it. To do it with you."

I laughed nervously. "You're a California kinda guy." David pumped up his chest. So, I thought, he liked being cool.

"Sounds good to me. Let's do it. Choose something from your list and I'll stand behind you so I can help you."

We both got up from our chairs and David stood closely behind me in the darkened room. I picked something frightening from my list. "I'm thinking of being in an airplane." Fear rumbled in my skull. "My head feels like it's going to explode."

"Here, I'll hold it together for a minute." David put his hands on my head and I could feel his fingers in my hair. I briefly thought of Richard. Then the doctor reached around me, took my hands and brought them up to my heart. Together we moved my hands from my chest out to my sides and back again. With every slow pump I took a deep gulp of air, filling myself with the fear of being in an airplane. Panic filled my body. Flames of terror licked my skin. It felt somehow familiar. David's breath was hot on the nape of my neck, his hands brushing against my chest with every pump. His hot body was now pressed against my back. A question flickered in my mind and quickly fizzled out: was that an erection? I couldn't think about it because I was now consumed completely by fear and it was time to flip the fear into love.

I stopped pumping and our hands rested together on my heart. I felt his thumb move closer to the swell of my breast. I was frightened by the intimacy and had to move things along. "Now I need to feel love fill my body." I was terrified and gasping for air. "I need to flip the fear into love."

I had experienced so much fear in my life, would this doctor actually turn it into love? I so wanted him to do this, even though I was unsure what "this" was and what it should feel like. His hands pressed hard on my heart, in between my breasts and I felt what I thought was a pure love enter me. Was it my imagination? Was this love? And how was David with all this? It mattered to me that I pleased him. He seemed so lost. Maybe he needed some positive reinforcement. I was so hardwired to take care of everyone that all I could think about was how to help him too.

"I can feel white light come from your hands into my heart," I whispered. "You are flipping the fear into love. I can feel it."

I stood completely still with his hands on my heart and willed myself to feel his white light expand through me like a warm glow. Was it love he was pouring into me?

It was time to test if the exercise had worked. "Now I'm imagining I'm in an airplane again." I stood still and waited for fear to consume me. Would it? I held my breath.

It didn't! Had this worked? I did a mental checklist of how I felt.

How had this happened so easily? Unbelievable!

I was ecstatic. The exercise had worked! I was no longer feeling the fear. I wasn't sure what I was feeling now, but perhaps it was love. "I'm okay. It worked, David! You helped me get rid of the fear! Thank you so much." Could I do anything with David's love in my heart? Yes! He *was* a good doctor.

He cleared his throat and said, "The exercise seemed to be success-ful, so we'll do it for the other items on your list. And maybe there are items that you didn't put on your list." David swept his arm around the room, "This room is a safe place for sex." He looked at me with a small smile playing around his eyes, eyebrows raised.

I gulped. It felt like I was swallowing ashes and they had stuck in my throat. What did he mean? Sex with him? No, he must mean I could talk about sex in this room. But why would I do that? Richard and I had a really fun and happy sexual relationship. We had some other problems, sure, like all married couples, but I was here because I needed help with anxiety.

He smiled at me. "You did good work today." He put his arms around me in a goodbye hug and pressed his hips against mine. He did have an erection!

"Thanks" I said as breezily as I could and quickly opened the office door, snapping on his office light as I made my hasty exit.

I sat in my car and hugged myself, waiting for the heater to stop the shaking deep inside my body. There was nothing wrong with him being turned on, was there? I decided it was okay. It was just a small bone of contention! I laughed right out loud as I turned on the ignition. I was so exhilarated. Or was I frightened? All the same, really, to me. I felt so alive! I decided I'd go back.

When I got home Richard was making dinner and the kids were doing their homework. I sat at the kitchen table and wrote the first poem I'd written in years and years. It was so different than textbooks. I felt guilty as I secretly ventured into a new sexual world that had nothing to do with Richard. I called the poem "Yes." It was about an orgasm. My heart constricted when I thought it was a good thing that Richard had his back turned as he was concocting his famous stew on the stove.

At my next appointment David turned out the light the minute I walked into his office. He asked me to tell him about my childhood and in the semi-darkness I tore the whole story out of my memory. The knives, the fire, the hitting, the poisoned pets, the underwear on the floor. My mother's death. It was awful to remember.

At the end of my session I said, "I've written a poem. The first one I've written in years. I like it, but I'm nervous about reading it to you." The shadows in the office seemed to slither around me and my birds were scrambling about in my head.

"Why?" he inquired.

"Well," I felt so immature, so awkward. "It's about an orgasm."

David raised himself out of his chair and leaned forward ominously, jutting out his chin. Suddenly he shouted, "Yeah? So?"

What? Why was he shouting? "*Yeah so? Yeah so?*" echoed in my ears as I sat there, dumbfounded. I hated shouting. It was second on my list of things I couldn't do: "Can't be shouted at." I rose to my feet unsteadily, turned on the light and muttered, "Bye."

I ran from his office in tears. My skin felt as if it were humming like a taut wire in the wind. It was my fault he'd shouted. It was my fault he was angry. I hadn't read him the poem. Maybe if I pleased him he wouldn't shout at me. I would go back and please him. I needed his help badly. He had helped me with the fear of flying. I would read the damn poem, no matter how nervous I was.

At my next appointment I broached the subject of the poem again. My heart was fluttering as I flattened the folded paper on my lap and my hands were damp and shaking. Spontaneously, I changed the title. I didn't want him to think I was agreeing to have sex with him. I loved my husband. There would be no "Yes" to other men.

I took a deep breath and began to read. My tongue stumbled over the sensual lines about the heaving, pulsing sea, but I made it to the end. I put the poem on my lap and looked up expectantly. I felt so electrified. Did he like it? He was just staring at me. My skin felt like it was blistering. He didn't say anything. Maybe silence was a thera-peutic strategy. But then he got up and announced we should work on 'flipping' another item on the list, elevators this time. Again, I felt his erection press against my bum as he stood behind me.

I was telling Ella how David was healing my anxiety by flipping my fear into love. How I could now do quite a few things on my list of impossible activities. I could get in an elevator. I could be on a balcony. I told her about his erections and I giggled like a schoolgirl.

Ella challenged me. "You call him David? Not Dr. Blackwood?"

"Yes, he told me to. He hugs me at the end of each appointment. We're partners."

"Are you sure what you're doing is therapy?"

"Well, now I can do almost everything that was on my list."

"What do you think of him?"

"I don't really know. His office is pretty skuzzy and I sort of want to clean it and take care of him; he seems so lost somehow. He wears the same pants every day. I feel all churned up and these powerful feelings keep coming over me. Everything feels so thrilling, almost frighteningly so. I feel so alive. Honestly, I think I might be in love with him."

"What about Richard?"

"I'm in love with him too, but with David it feels so exhilarating, it gets my adrenaline going! I think I must be head over heels in love with him."

I worked on my anxiety list with David over the next few weeks, but I really wasn't feeling that well. I had a constant stomach ache. I mentioned it to David and he decided to do an internal examination on me. As David was taking off the thin latex gloves he said, "I've noticed that you seem quite upset these days and I think your stomach problems are from your general anxiety," he declared. "It's not unusual for patients to go to therapy appointments twice, or even three times a week."

I pulled up my pants while he jotted in my file. It felt odd to have my therapist's fingers inside me. I liked it, sort of, or I thought I did, but it didn't matter really what I thought, did it? He was helping me and he knew what was best for me. But I felt guilty. Was this cheating on Richard? I wasn't like that. I loved Richard. Well, it was just an internal and he was a doctor, after all. I knew what was *really* bothering me. The Coroner's Report. I hadn't been able to stop thinking about it.

"Oh, you think I should see you more often?"

"I think it would help. Why don't you come twice a week."

At the end of the session he held his arms open to hug me. We'd already had several goodbye hugs, all seemingly perfunctory and polite, if only from the waist up. Sometimes he was turned on and sometimes he wasn't. But this time, his cheek caressed mine so slowly I felt he was rocking my soul and making love to me. Did doctors hug their patients like this? Was this love? I was so confused. On my way out I made an appointment for later in the week.

That night I went into my office with a beer. I didn't want Richard to see me drinking and writing a poem to David. As I drank I remembered over and over again how his cheek had felt, pressed against mine. It felt as if our souls were merging and melting, sinking and floating together, as if our inner galaxies were swirling together in a primordial rocking, swaying back and forth, like he was making love to me. We had connected together. It felt almost religious. I wrote it all down in a poem and called it, "Cheek Against Cheek." I wasn't great at titles.

Two days later, at my new second "regular" weekly appointment, I read it to him. Again he said nothing. But he didn't dispute what I was saying about him in the poem. Did that mean he loved me? And I must have been pleasing him because he didn't shout at me. Again he just stared at me after I finished reading. It was awkward.

I looked away and fidgeted with my purse. I was trying to get up my courage to talk about the Coroner's Report.

Finally he demanded, "What is it?"

I started babbling, "I never knew how my mother died so I wrote to the Coroner. I can't understand the report. Although the verdict was suicide, I don't know if it was accidental or deliberate. Did she take handfuls of pills? I can't understand the measurements. I also don't know if there was a complete police investigation; she had cuts and bruises on her body and I think she could have been murdered." I whispered the word.

"Why don't you bring in the Report and I'll have a look at it."

That was so nice of him! Two days later David sat closely beside me and held the Coroner's Report on his knee so I could see it. I had practically thrown it at him because I didn't want to touch it. He explained as much as he could, but he didn't know what the figures meant either.

"Don't worry," he reassured me. "I know where to call to get the info."

David would help me! "Thank you," I told him. "I really appreciate it. I really should know how my mother died, After all, I'm forty-one now. I think I can handle it."

He gave me quite a long hug before I turned on the ceiling fan light and left. He always turned it out for our sessions. And I always turned it on when I left. I still didn't like the dark, but that ceiling fan drove me nuts. Why didn't he just turn off the bloody fan and leave the light on? Oh well, he was just trying to be thoughtful. It was a loving gesture, really. I was grateful he was being so kind. I knew I was pleasing him now. He was being really nice to me.

CHAPTER 4

M Y APPOINTMENTS WITH DAVID came and went in the darkened room while he and I talked more about my childhood abuse. David discussed with me how this would have an impact on my sexuality and he decided that my sexual wires, so to speak, were now malfunctioning.

He looked at me earnestly. "Naturally, anyone who went through what you went through as a child would have impaired sexuality. Do you have any problems along that line?"

I was non-committal and swallowed an embarrassed reply.

"Thought so," he said. "Your sexual 'wires', so to speak, are probably not functioning properly. It would help if you were 'rewired'."

"Rewired." I repeated. What on earth did he have in mind? How could a person's sexuality be rewired?

David explained that through touch we could create healthy new pathways of pleasure from my erogenous zones to my core. To get around the rules of the College of Physicians and Surgeons, which stated that doctors couldn't sexually touch their patients, David created a "contract" for the rewirings. It was agreed that *I* would guide his hand over my body thus removing him from any active involvement.

How did I feel about all this sudden sexual activity? I felt like crying. I loved the way my husband touched me. I had no idea I was so sexually screwed up, but of course David was right. And I was grateful that he would help me with my problems. He was going out of his way to be kind to me and I wanted to be a good patient and get better. Was I upset or was I thrilled? I didn't know how I felt. I felt the way I had always felt. My emotions were whirring together in a chaotic ball, as usual. But one thing I knew for sure, I wanted to feel better.

So now David was "rewiring" me. With his rules in place, he stood behind me and gave me his hand. I guided his fingers across my lips. But wait, I could smell carbon on them. Had he been masturbating before my appointment? And was that another erection? Alarm, disgust, and attraction all whirled through me. I could hear him breathing raggedly behind my back. Should I refuse to go on? No, we were doing an *exercise*. It was legit. He was helping me. And he might shout at me. I didn't want that.

I guided his fingertips over my eyes, nose, neck, and then down to my breasts, nipples, and belly, to finally land on my clitoris. His middle finger stimulated me but I knew it was a wasted effort. My emotions were churning. I was frightened, although I didn't know why. An image of Richard flew across my mind and a pain squeezed my heart. But I wanted David to feel good. He seemed like such a sad man. I wanted to please him so badly. I wanted him to love me, to not be angry at me. To not hurt me. So I faked it.

When the rewiring was "complete," at least in David's mind, he went to his chair, a little smile on his face, and I went to mine. Good, he felt better about himself. He crossed his legs and covered his crotch. But what was he doing with his hands? Was he trying to hide his thumbs as he rubbed himself with them?

I felt nauseous and looked out the filmy window to avoid looking at his moving hands. I said, "I am very grateful you are helping me like this, considering."

"Considering what?" he asked.

"Considering I'm an ugly piece of shit." Like duh, didn't he know that?

"I see we have a ways to go."

"Oh. Well, now I have to go. That's what therapy's like. Comings and goings," I laughed. He didn't get the joke.

That night I was on autopilot getting dinner for the family, making sure the kids' homework was done, and talking with Richard about his day at work. While watching TV with the family I replayed in my mind the rewiring event. My anxiety about what it meant was overshadowed by the memory of David holding me. It felt as if soft warm water was cascading from his arms and I was swimming in his love as he touched me. I could feel the slow white heat from his erection smoking up into me, turning his love into steam and melting the two of us in a circle of fire. I felt anchored in that circle and I truly believed that he thought I was a beautiful woman. My heart swelled with gratitude because I believed, deep, deep down, that I was an ugly piece of shit. Maybe this could change. I grabbed the pad of paper beside me and wrote "The Making of a Beautiful Woman" at the top.

"What are you writing, honey?" Richard asked during a commercial.

I covered the paper with my hand, I felt so guilty. "Oh, nothing sweetie, just a shopping list for tomorrow." What was I doing?

Later, after Richard had gone out for his walk, I grabbed not one but two beers and went into my office. The rewirings were magical. When David stood behind me, his touch in the silence was so profound I could hear his blood listening to mine, I could feel passion ricocheting between us and exploding into swirling flames, causing an implosion of the universe as it spun. I felt we were in a deep, breathing purple sea of home. Was I in love with him? I was something, that's for sure.

I felt spellbound, that was it. Spellbound.

I knew his sign was Cancer and that Cancers craved a steady home life. I wrote at the top of the page, "Home." I thought he'd like the pun at the end about coming home. Perhaps he would get it this time.

Weeks and weeks went by and we filled his dark office with rewirings, tears, and long hugs. I daydreamed about the rewiring sessions and remembered how quiet they were. How I could hear nothing but the sound of his touch on my body. How his hands were flaming hot as they ignited the arch of my back. How his touch sent crackling sparks into my core. He was outside me and entering in. I wrote about all this as I relived the sound of the fire dancing between us as his hands burned over every inch of my skin. I wrote a poem called "Listening to Fire."

I hid all the poems I wrote in my sock drawer. I now had a terrible secret from Richard. As I tugged the drawer open every night I felt as if an open wound in my heart was being rubbed with salt. I felt as if my mind was trapped in a cave. After writing each poem I rocked back and forth in my cold, dark office, bundled in my blue sleeping bag and whispering to myself. I stared at the black mirror of my window, hypnotized by my reflection, by the tears streaming down my face. I felt as if my head would explode. I could hear the wings of fear beating against the sides of my skull.

The birds were having a heyday.

Why was this happening? How could I stop it? I had gone to a doc-

tor for help and now I seemed so much worse. But I had to go back
to him. I just had to. I must be in love with him. And he went way
beyond the line of duty and rewired me. Was this because he loved me?
Must be. I was desperate to feel like myself again and I had no other
options. Also, if I stopped going he would be hurt and I wouldn't be
able to bear that. And deep down, I knew I deserved to feel the way I
did. I found a strange comfort in the familiarity of the pain, of being
bad. He'd said the healing process would not be easy.

After several rewirings I was up to five or six beers a night and I'd
drink them one after the other. I started whispering sentences into the
dark as I rocked, "And then the man turned me on. And then the man
pressed his erection against my bum. And then the man wanted me
to come. And then the man ... what did the man do? And then the
man sodomized me, that's what the man did. He hurt me." *Who is
the man? Who is the man?* I would cry and cry, "Who is the man?"
After drinking more, I would start my whispering chant all over again.
"*And then the man and then the man.*" Night after night for what
seemed to be an eternity I rocked back and forth huddled in the dark,
whispering to myself.

Every night Richard would look in and say, "It's time for us to go to
bed honey, it's late." And I would hide my face from him. I was in such
pain because of what I was doing and my heart felt like it was being
ripped apart. I was ashamed of being in such a state. I'd listen to his
footsteps receding down the hall and begin my chant again. Eventually
I'd stagger into the bedroom and crawl into bed beside him, shivering,
trying not to touch him with my cold body. I'd fall asleep with only
David in my head.

"What's going on with me David? I seem worse."

"You are having a healing crisis. It's a normal part of the therapy
process."

"But who is the man, David?"

"You are having very intense flashbacks of your childhood. This is the
work you need to do. The man is someone from your childhood."

"Like who? A teacher? I can't think of a teacher doing this to me.
My older brother certainly didn't. Sure he hurt me, but that wasn't
his fault. It couldn't have been my uncle—I never saw him. Who is
the man, David?"

"He must be your father. There's nobody else it could be." I tried to absorb this information. *My father?* My father didn't hurt me. *Did he?*

"I don't believe it."

David looked at me disapprovingly. "This is a very difficult time for you. I've noticed you seem apologetic about making extra appointments. I want you to feel free to come in any time."

I tucked this away into the back of my mind. He wanted to see me more often. He did love me.

"We can act out what your father did to you in a month or so. When you're ready."

He held me so softly before I left. I loved everything about him. No one had been this kind to me. He was helping me so much. I ran my hands up and down his back and felt the muscles in his bum. I whispered into his chest, "I know I keep asking, but I am desperate to know. Have you heard from the Coroner's Office? Can you tell me if my mother took handfuls of pills? Was it an accident?"

"They haven't returned my call."

I was more than disappointed. "Maybe you should call again. It's been ages." I could be disapproving, too.

I turned on the office light and left. I sat in the car and touched where his cheek had been on my face. He loved me. I tried to stop shaking.

I turned the key in the ignition. *Did he love me? Of course he did.* What was I going to make for dinner? Omelets? *Of course he loved me.* And Emma had that project due on Africa. *He loved me.* I needed to get her Bristol board. Shopper's Drug Mart. I backed the car out. *Right, Kathy, onward ho. Get a grip.*

Funny that in his office David always used my girlhood name, even though I told him my friends called me Sky. Well, I guess it made sense because Kathryn was the name on my insurance card, but it had been a long time since I'd thought of myself as Kathy.

I sat in front of David and laughed, "You won't believe this."

I reached into my purse. I had decided to tell him how I felt birds' wings fluttering in my head. I had even figured out that it happened when I got frightened or humiliated. I had drawn a picture of one of the birds; it looked like an Escher raven. I had drawn it with black ink on a black piece of construction paper.

I looked him straight in the eye. "I have birds in my head."

I watched him carefully. He didn't laugh. "I got them the night of my mother's funeral when I was fifteen."

I was speaking so fast. What was happening to me? The room felt unsteady and had become a sepia colour. "And now whenever I get upset I can hear them. I told Catherine Thorne, my therapist friend out east, about them and that I wanted to kill them. She said, 'no, don't do that, they're doing a job.' She said the birds would go away if I just talked to them and found out what their job was. They look like this." I thrust the paper at him.

He took it and held it up to the gray light coming through the window so he could see the black birds on the black paper. "So, you have to talk to the birds. Seems like a plan. How do I fit in?"

"The birds of fear, that's what I call them, the birds of fear live in a cave on the right side of my head. Right here." I tapped my skull about two inches above my ear. I could hear the thumps of my fingers inside my ear. "Maybe after I find out what their job is you could hold me and pump your white light of love through me up into the cave so they'll just melt away."

"I think I could do that."

"Thank you for not laughing at me."

"Why would I laugh?" He seemed genuinely puzzled.

Was he stupid?

"Oh David, for heaven's sake, it's not the done thing to have birds in your head. Get real." We both burst out laughing.

So David put his hands on my back while I talked to my birds and asked them what their job was. They said it was to keep me safe! Then his hands pumped his white light of love into my back and up into my brain, melting the birds away. The birds were gone.

Now I had David in my head, my lovely David. *He* would keep me safe. I knew how I really felt now, no question.

I was totally in love with him.

CHAPTER 5

A MONTH WENT BY and David believed that I was ready to start acting out some of the things that had happened to me as a child and that this would help me cope with the memories. That's why I was now lying on David's office floor pretending to be asleep, remembering how I felt years ago at the age of eleven, lying in my bed. A white hiss of sound was building at the edges of my mind. The unwritten script was from those nights in my childhood when I heard creaks on the stairs and then I disappeared into TV snow, the nights when my pink underwear ended up on the floor of my bedroom and I didn't know why.

The office was a hazy black except for a white band of light coming from the gap under the door. David had shut the venetian blinds and the overhead lights were turned off as usual. He was outside in the hall. Through my half-closed eyelids I could see the toes of his shoes under the door. He was acting out the role of my father. *The man.*

As David opened the office door, his body was silhouetted against the square of light. He shut the door softly and kneeled beside me. He pretended to take off my pink underwear, tugging with clenched fists in a pantomimed struggle with the panties and then, once successful, threw them on the floor beside me. David inched along the carpet to my feet and then spread my knees, crawling between them. He opened my legs wider, ran his hands over my breasts, and put his mouth just over my crotch. His teeth opened and his tongue flicked in the air.

I looked down my body and watched, frozen in horror, as the light from under the door crept up his face, creating ghostly shadows as he licked the air. Spaces in his lower teeth made him look like a lion devouring me. The design on the wall hanging behind him shimmered and danced, its deep blood red colour spreading across the black wall. A white crackle of fear hummed like static in my ears and wild screams echoed in my head.

Terror fired through my veins. "Stop. David, stop!" I could hardly breathe. I felt I was drowning underwater.

His shadowy bulk leaned back and I thought he was going to pounce on me. I could see his eyes glittering through the darkness and another silent scream swelled inside my chest and burst into my brain. Suddenly his shape turned and in the band of light I could see him circling away, crawling on his hands and knees to sit at the front of the examination table. He opened his arms and legs wide and gestured for me to come to him. I scrambled between his legs and rested against his chest, sobbing. Somewhere in the back of my mind I registered that he was aroused.

I shivered, "Are you sure this is good therapy?" I felt so cold.

His voice was calming. "I know someone who works with adolescents and he said that role playing events is a well known therapy treatment. We'll keep at it until you can be calm while you do it. Until you can face what your father did to you."

Was it my father? Really? I tried to remember exactly what had happened, way back when, but my mind seemed to be blocked by a roar of static electricity.

"Maybe next time will be easier," said David encouragingly.

I rested in his arms while I waited for the fear to seep out of my body. I was so grateful he was taking good care of me. My skin was buzzing with what felt like electrical current. I was so in love with him. And I knew he loved me. The fact that we were in love was the one thing that kept me going in what was now a life of chaos. I felt as if I had fallen into a deep dark underwater cave and his love for me was a lifeline.

We had our usual goodbye hug, I turned on the light and then, when I got to my car, I read my written list of what I had to do that day for my children. I picked up Jamie from school and took him to baseball. I went to the grocery store to buy Cheerios. I drove like a robot. I would not fail my children.

That night, after cleaning up the hard, sticky mess from the pan of honey garlic chicken wings, I turned on the light in my office, lined up six beers in front of me and wrote the first of many poems about caves. I didn't really know what they were about, but I knew I was gripped with fear as I wrote them. I wrote about a lion pacing around me and an open, bleeding wound in my belly. I licked the wound and hated the tasted of blood. I tried to escape, but couldn't. The cave floor was full of blood red paw prints. I didn't know what the poems meant;

they came from a deep, indescribable, instinctual place. Even though I refused to act out the underwear scene again, a few weeks later David suggested that I was now ready to act out a mini drama about how my father had sodomized me. We called it "Flip the Flip."

We decided it would start with David playing the role of my father and holding me facing him while I described how my father had sexually stimulated me. Then I would be turned around, or "flipped" so to speak, and punished with a vicious anal rape because I had become turned on. And then I would be spun back to face David, who would help flip the bad experience into a good one. Then I would be spun around yet again, so my back was to David, who would rewire me, flipping the bad sex with my father into good sex with David.

We faced each other in the dark, our arms around each other. I murmured into David's ear how my father had turned me on and then how he had to punish me for being aroused by raping me anally. David's arms circled me while I turned to put my back to him. I could feel his erection pressing against me. I was terrified. I was in love. I was thrilled. I was underwater. My heart thumped chaotically in my ears.

I despaired. *What the fuck were we doing? Why were we doing it?*

I described the rape. "And then he put his hand over my mouth so I couldn't scream." My mind was jumping around. Was all this true? But David loosely covered my mouth with his right hand. Panic rose in me but I persevered to please him.

"And then he held me tightly around my neck so I would choke if I tried to get away." I could feel the hair on David's skin brush against my face as he put his left arm across my neck. His right hand was now sweaty as it grazed my lips when I talked. "And then he would play with me some more until I felt I was about to have an orgasm. And then he would say to me, 'This is what you deserve.'" As I described how the man had sodomized me, David pressed his erection against me.

I whispered into the dark, "There David, that was the flip. Now we have to flip the bad experience into a good one. We have to flip the flip." I felt like I was going to faint, but David's arms held me upright. I slowly spun back towards him in his arms, giving physical meaning to the word "flip." Facing him, I whispered into his chest, "I can see you rescuing me from my father." I told David what I saw in my mind's eye. "You are throwing my father off of me and chopping him into a thousand pieces. You have saved me."

I then turned around again in David's arms to finish flipping the flip. I put my back to him and he gave me his hand so I could guide it over my erogenous zones, as we had done when he was rewiring me. His middle finger stimulated me so that I could have an orgasm, therefore completing the final flip. But I was frightened by the rape scene and couldn't focus on the pleasure he was trying to give me. But I loved David so much, I had to make him feel he was a good lover, so again I pretended to have an orgasm.

"There David, we flipped the flip. The bad sex has been replaced with good sex." I loved him. It felt like my body was vibrating in the dark.

David held me tightly. "We'll do it several times to make sure you're healed. You did good work today."

I said, "I couldn't have done it without my spin doctor."

I felt David's laugh chortling deep in his chest while we stood silently together in the dark, his arms around me. I loved our goodbye hugs.

Now during our farewell embraces, I often touched him and today I ran my finger slowly like a river down the valley of his spine. I felt my touch was a soft breeze that sighed through the downy hair on the back of his head. I reached down and touched the inside of his legs and then moved up to feel his nipples. I felt I was stroking him like the fire of a sunset. Tonight I would write a poem about touching him, with the theme of earth, fire, air, and water. I would read it to him tomorrow. I could already see him listening, his hands cupped over his groin, thumbs down, his legs tightly crossed. This is how it always was. He loved me. I knew that much. And I was reeling in love with him. I pecked him on the cheek, turned on the light and left.

"You're looking so pretty, Mommy, you seem different." Margaret was watching me adoringly while the family was eating dinner.

"Thanks honey... here, have some salad."

"Mommies always look beautiful to their kids," said Richard, looking at me appraisingly.

Could Richard tell what was going on with David and me?

That night, after the kids were in bed and Richard was out with a buddy, I put seven beers on my desk and a new pad of paper under my light. What would I write? Earth, fire, air and water. Hmmm. How I was being deeply loved by David? I caressed the pad and remembered how I had lain on the earth years ago, feeling my soul seep into the universe. How I had received the loving interconnectedness of everything. How this had filled me with a deep inner peace. David made me feel as if I were completely loved, just as I had been loved by the universe that night under the stars. I stared off into space and then began to write furiously. David and I were ebbing and flowing together through everything that existed. I imagined his arms around me and recaptured the same feeling of peace that had blanketed me years ago. As long as I had David flooding through me, I would be safe. I accepted the feeling and became one with the breathtakingly beautiful landscape of him.

After flipping the flip about six times I felt like I was falling apart. I wept and wept in David's arms and only survived the therapy because his love flowed through me and consumed my fear. But as the horror of what my father had done to me sank in, my whole world outside David's office seemed to disintegrate. How could my dad have betrayed me like this? It didn't make any sense. *My dad? Who I loved?* All the physical abuses from Lynny-poo and my brother and now *this?* Was it true? David said it was. It must be. He was my doctor.

I felt I was made of frozen, fragile glass and swimming underwater. I was watching myself break into tiny shards of ice. I needed David to hold me together softly so I could heal while I tried to exist, to be. I was having trouble living, even on autopilot. Giving my children the semblance of a normal life was taking every ounce of my effort. I could no longer read the newspaper or watch TV. Everything I looked at was shaded a deep sepia, the colour of faded photographs. My skin seemed to be cold and brittle. Corners of rooms were crazily askew and shifted in and out of focus. It felt like my limbs kept disappearing and reappearing. I felt as if I were underneath the ocean surf, being tumbled about and whacked against rocks.

"Is this a healing crisis?" Even though I was sitting still in front of David, I felt like I was losing my balance. David was poking his glasses up his nose.

"I think so. This often happens in therapy."

"I feel like I'm underwater and I'll never surface. I feel like a Picasso woman living in a Van Gogh painting. Everything keeps shifting on me. I can't read."

"Have you had your eyes checked lately?"

I almost cried. Sometimes he was so stupid! But I was now utterly dependent upon David to save me from drowning, from shattering apart, to save me from the crooked rooms were the corners didn't meet. I needed him to keep me safe because my birds were gone. He had melted them away with his white light of love and he was in my head instead. We were one. I had to keep going back to see him, otherwise I'd die. I had no choice.

While I was in his arms during our long goodbye hug, I imagined that he was skating on a frozen lake while I swam below him, trapped under the ice. I could hear the sharp edge of his metal blades carving around and around above me as he skated. As he fell in love with me, he fell down, breaking through the weakened ice.

When he saw me swimming below the ice, he dove down and carried me gently to the surface. The heat from his hands was like a blanket on my body and melted the water that had frozen all around me. The ice tinkled like falling fairy dust as it disappeared. And then we swam happily together in the lovely water while the waves swam in us. The way David was rescuing me felt like magic. It was magic. I was in his spell.

I rested my head against his chest as he held me before I left his office. I had to keep seeing him. It was my only hope. I turned on the light and waved as merrily as I could at Lydia as I swam past the waiting room.

Richard was in the kitchen stretching for his evening march through the neighbourhood. As he lifted his arms over his head I could see his mouth was an angry slash. "Sky, you're being so curt with me. And impatient with the kids. And you're drinking too much. It's like I don't know you anymore. I miss my fun wife."

"Oh Richard, of course I love you. It's just that I am working so hard at my therapy."

"Like what?"

I took a deep breath. "My father sexually abused me, Richard. That's what."

"Your Dad? I don't believe it."

"Oh believe it, alright. David helped me remember it all."

"How'd he help you?" Richard had stopped stretching and stood motionless, glaring at me.

"He told me."

"Well, he told you wrong. Your father did no such thing." Richard's angry face seemed to float in and out of focus.

"David Blackwood's a *doctor*. I believe him." *Didn't I?*

Richard turned on his heel and stamped out of the kitchen into the dark. I opened the fridge door and loaded myself up with beers. They clunked together as I floated up the stairs to my office. I was going to write a poem called "The Frozen Lake."

CHAPTER 6

To HEAL THE SCARS of my childhood abuse, David and I devised a treatment called body scans. Before we started doing the scans, David created a contract so he would be operating within the College's rules. I was to be fully clothed as I lay on the examination table and I was to guide David's hand to touch the parts of my body that had been harmed. He would then heal them with what had quickly become his famous "white light of love." We had done numerous scans over the course of several months that all involved him touching my breasts and between my legs. I loved the way he touched me.

David gave me his hand and I placed his fingertips on my temple. "This is where my brother hit me with a golf club." He rubbed my temple and through his touch I could feel his love caress my skin.

"This is where the point of Lynn's knife nicked my skin when she cut my sweater off." His fingertips stroked between my breasts.

"These are the breasts Lynn laughed at." His fingers played around and around my breasts. Our eyes were locked, his sparkling through his eyelashes as he looked down at me in the dim light. I felt somehow frightened. No, I was excited. I got it wrong.

I put his finger between my legs and could feel him touch me under the thin material of my skirt. "This is what my father touched." *Was it my father?*

As I moved his finger he withdrew his hand and said, "You do that."

My heart froze. What was this? "But you've always done it. What's up?" I glanced at his crotch. He was usually aroused by now.

"I'm not comfortable with doing that anymore." He spit out his words.

"Please don't be mad at me," I begged. Would he shout? "We negotiated that in a contract. It was to be me guiding your hand so it would be my energy, not yours. Me. Not you. Remember? So that everything that happened in here would be my fault. Don't be mad."

He patted the head of the table. "Go ahead, you won't be alone. I will be with you in a very powerful way."

"That's okay." I swung my legs off the table and stepped down onto his stool. I felt my heart had been stabbed with a knife. I had disappointed him. I needed to get away before either he shouted or I cried.

"It's time for me to go anyway."

How many times had he put his finger on me? All those rewirings. All those scans. And now he wouldn't? Why not? Was I an ugly piece of shit after all? Didn't he love me anymore? How humiliating to ask for something and be rejected like that. Pain bled into my chest. But I wasn't going to show it. Oh no, I had my pride.

I tossed him a lop-sided smile, gave him a perfunctory hug and snapped on the light. "See ya." I adjusted my top as I tried to slink away.

I cooked up a storm for my family, vegetarian casserole, salad, home-made rolls, the works. While the dish bubbled in the oven, I stewed. Then there was the routine of clearing up the dishes, making lunches, doing homework, kissing the kids goodnight and finally chatting with Richard for a bit. After he left for his nightly walk I went upstairs to my office with eight beers clinking together in a shopping bag while my thoughts clunked together in my skull. Before the office door was even shut I began to cry.

I drank and drank. He didn't love me. He hated touching me. I felt utterly humiliated, like I was in an underwater nightmare. I wrote about fish. How I felt like the white underbelly of my soul was floating face up in the moonlight waiting for David to claw me. About how frightened I was, darting to the edges of a glass barrier, trying to get away but hitting it with my mouth gaping wide, wanting to scream but only making the strangled non-sounds one makes in a nightmare. How terror and pain filled me when he hooked me with his claws, spread my legs, and told me that I smelled like fish. I called the poem "Fish."

I tiptoed into my bedroom as quietly as I could, but Richard woke up. He got so angry when we didn't fall asleep in each other's arms, the way we used to.

"It's late! Come to bed sooner." He turned over, exhaling angrily.

"Sorry honey." I slid the poem into my drawer under all the others, careful to not make any shuffling noises that would tip Richard off that I was hiding something under my socks. I climbed into bed as quietly as I could and stared at the ceiling. I'd never read the poem to David. And I hoped Richard never saw it.

I pulled the blankets up to my chin. I reached for Richard in the dark, a pain ricocheting in my chest.

"Trust our relationship," David was saying to me. "I know it's hard, but just trust the relationship. I know your parenting was substandard."

I started to cry and cry. Memories of my childhood tumbled around in my brain. Lynn and knives, asthma and dead pets, my poor knee, the scars all over my body, my living with the constant fear that I would be killed.

David looked at me softly. "I could hold you like a parent holds a child. Re-parent you. Cradle you. It would be your medicine for anxiety. You could learn how to trust."

"I'll take my medicine," I sobbed.

He got out of his chair and sat down with his back against the examination table. He spread his legs, revealing a white thread hanging from the seam of his pants at the crotch. He opened his arms and gestured for me to sit on his lap, as if he were a big comfy chair. I sank down onto his chest, his knees spread on either side of me. I tried to calm the fear beating inside my heart. Why was I so afraid? I imagined myself being his little girl and him being a kind, loving daddy. I could feel his love for me as he gently wrapped his arms around me and rested his hands on my chest. Through my jangled nerves I registered his erection against my back.

"I'm terrified."

"Hmmm. It's okay." He stroked my hair.

His voice was so soothing and consoled my tears. I was exhausted and rested my soul in his. I knew he loved me. I trusted him completely. I curled up against him and waited for the sobs to stop shuddering through my body.

Finally I lay there quietly and imagined I could hear music echoing back and forth off our bones and souls like waves of water moving back and forth in crests and crescendos. As we melted into each other, the water became mirror flat and our two songs floated together in a perfect reflection of harmony. I could hear us breathing quietly together as I listened to the song become quiet. Eventually it became so pure it made no sound at all. There was a silence between us, a silence of peace and love and happiness. I trusted him with all my heart as I lay in his arms. I knew I was listening to the song of all songs. I knew the song of songs could only happen to lovers. I knew we were lovers. I was sure of that. I would write a poem tonight called "The Song of Songs."

David and I were just finishing up a body scan where yet again we had followed the rules. I was lying down as I guided his hand over my heart so he could fill it with his white light of love and heal it from the pain caused by my mother's death.

David's voice penetrated my tears. "I heard from the Coroner's Office."

What had he said? The Coroner? "Oh?"

Fear prickled at my skin. What was David going to tell me? "Did she take handfuls?" I shut my eyes, bracing myself for the answer.

"Handfuls." He stroked my breast.

"I'm so glad you're the one telling me." So it wasn't murder. It was suicide. *Was it really?* Blackness settled over me like a veil. "I feel like I'm dying. Please fill me with your white light of love."

"I feel you've given me the power to heal you."

"You are healing me," I said as the energy from his hands flowed into me.

"Why do I have this power?"

"I don't know David. You just do. Doctors have power. And I'm just grateful you are using it to save me." *But what about the gash on her lip? Her swollen eye?*

"I love you," he said.

The words whispered into my soul.

David was going away for his summer holidays. Three long weeks. Would I survive? Would he? I was dashing up to his office virtually every day for at least a hug. I just had to be touched by him. It was a need, like eating. I believed he needed me too because before he left, David decided he would teach me foreplay.

I lay on my back and David gave me his hand. We started out following our contract rules as I guided his hot fingertips over my body. But then he continued the fiery journey on his own down to places I couldn't reach. He seared the skin between my thighs, set my knees alight and softly flamed his fingers around my ankles.

Once he had set the front of me on fire he told me to turn over. I grunted as I heaved myself onto my belly. I had become so fat from drinking that I felt like a whale flopping on a beach. I laughed.

"Okay, okay, I know, I'm fat. Forty-two year olds get fat. While you're away, I'll go on a diet." He didn't respond. "Oh no, have I destroyed the atmosphere?"

"No, no, we're fine," he said as his touch smouldered at the nape of my neck. His hands slowly burned down my back, smoked over my buttocks, and then ignited the crease behind my knee. And then he stopped, leaving me blazing like a bonfire on his examination table.

"Oh. Wow." I said, jiggling over onto my back. "Wow. Have you ever taught me foreplay." My body was a spark away from complete combustion.

He looked at his watch and then at me. My hour was up. And so was he.

"Three weeks." I sighed. "I'm worried I won't survive without you."

"Here," he held out his hand, "give me your necklace."

Mystified, I sat up on the examination table and handed it to him. He curled his fingers slowly around it. Then he shut his eyes and bowed his head, his fist held tight against his chest. While his eyes were closed I looked at his crotch. Yup, that was a bulge alright.

"There," he smiled as he handed it back. "I will be with you while we are apart."

It was magic.

When I got into my car I turned on the air conditioning full blast.

CHAPTER 7

WHILE DAVID WAS AWAY, hot love poems flowed out of my pen like lava. And now he was finally back! But I was running late for my appointment and drove madly to his office, bending over the car's air conditioning to fluff my damp hair. The poems for him were steaming in my purse. I raced into the waiting room and caught my breath.

Suddenly there he was, my lovely David! Good looking and tanned in his pale blue oxford cloth shirt and ... the same old pants.

Why didn't his wife take better care of him? *I would*, I thought. I would make sure he looked great. This morning Richard had worn the black suit with the silvery gray tie. He'd looked so handsome leaving the house with the lunch I'd made for him.

David looked up from the file he was carrying and our eyes met. My heart pounded in my ears like surf on rocks. "Kathy."

I almost swooned. I stood up and felt my body being pulled towards his, like water following a full moon. I sat on the edge of my chair, grinning from ear to ear. "Well? Tell me, how was it? Your trip I mean?"

"Fine, but the focus is on you."

What's this? He was being so distant. He sounded like a *doctor*. I babbled, "I've written you some poems. In fact, I wrote to you every day you were gone. Do you want to read them?" I held the smoking bundle out to him.

He was being so stiff. And not in the right places. He took my poems and put them in his desk drawer without a glance. I was stunned, confused, and hastily made an excuse about being late for an appointment. I had to get out of there.

At my next appointment, David reached into his desk drawer. "Here's the letter you wrote me. I'm catching up still from my holiday and I don't have time to read anything extra."

Pain curled around my heart. *Letter?* They were *love* poems. I put them back into my purse. Oh no, now what was he saying?

"I don't feel sexual towards you."

I felt shattered. "But you just taught me foreplay. That was pretty sexual."

"Well, maybe for *you*."

As if he hadn't been there! Suddenly I had a flash of understanding. "Look, if you're worried I'll report you, I won't. I love you, David. And I know you love me. That's why you want to help me. Please don't worry. It's me guiding your hand. That was our deal, remember, so you wouldn't get in trouble. My hand moving yours. Well, except for that business behind my knee," I laughed. He didn't.

"I am not sexually involved with you."

I burst into tears, "But I thought you loved me."

"Like a parent loves a child." He pursed his lips and stared at me.

It was all too much. But he *always* had an erection when he held me "like a child."

From foreplay to a cover story? It was time to blow his cover. Two could play at this game. I sobbed, "Oh please, hold me. I need some medicine. Please?"

Finally David relented, got down on the floor, and spread his legs for me to sit between. His arm rested across my chest and I could see its soft downy hair flutter as I breathed. And there it was, his erection, pressing into my back like a steel rod.

"David?" I waited for his soft grunt to make sure he was listening. It was now or never. I gathered up all my courage. "David? Do you have an erection?"

"No. No, I don't." He shifted his body under me, trying to hide it. "But our time's up. Have you had enough medicine?"

I looked at my watch as I got off his lap. Time wasn't up, he was. But my whole body was shaking. I hadn't had enough medicine. "David, I feel like my arms are disappearing and the room keeps shifting its shape."

He stood up. "I'll prescribe you a drug for anxiety called Ativan."

So, he wasn't going to hug me on the floor anymore today, probably because I had noticed he was turned on and he had to get back at me. He knew I hated taking drugs.

"Ativan? I can't take anything addictive. Is it addictive?"

"No, not at all. I take it. It's a good drug. And it wears off fast."

Why was he being so mean to me? Why couldn't he just admit that he loved me sexually? Was he frightened of true love? Or was it because he was supposed to be professionally detached? Maybe it was both.

He sat in his chair beside his desk to write the prescription. His legs were spread and one hand nonchalantly rested over himself. Did he think he could hide it? I saw that dumb white thread hanging from the inner seam of his crotch. Should I tell him about the thread? No, better not, then he'd know I'd been looking. Why did nobody take care of him? No wonder he takes Ativan. Smokes dope too. I remembered when I asked him if he smoked and he'd said, "I smoke dope." Maybe that's why his behaviour was so erratic. He handed the prescription to me.

Before going to the grocery store to get Richard some coffee, I stopped off at the library and looked up Ativan. What? It *was* addictive. I felt betrayed. I crumpled the prescription into a wad and took some deep breaths.

But we moved on. Appointments went by. Periodically David acted out raping me in the dark. Periodically he scanned me from head to toe. Periodically I could feel my soul being cradled as he hugged me. Periodically I heard the song of songs, the singing silence of nothingness between us. And I always felt his hand touching me like the soft curl of a wave frothing on a sandy beach. I always felt as if I was swimming in his foam. I told him I loved him. Every now and then he told me he loved me. I held on to those moments like a drowning woman in a lifeboat.

I took Jamie and Margaret to Lake Placid in the Adirondacks for their March Break. While I talked with my kids, I only thought of David. David had become the landscape of my soul where my god used to be.

As I lay in my Holiday Inn bed, with Margaret and Jamie safely tucked in a bed beside mine, I thought of how I was one with David as I listened to the wind gliding down the sides of the mountains. And because David had been so sexual with me, my god in nature had become sexual. The wind sounded like a hand caressing a scantily clad woman, rustling over forests and rocks. The breath of the wind kissed the brooks and licked deep into the valleys. I could hear the Adirondacks moaning with the pleasure of the wind as it slowly slid its hand under the skirt of the forest. The fingers of breeze played with the foam on the rivers until the mountains leaned into the rising wind and everything gripped and throbbed.

David was now so deeply embedded in my psyche that I thought I was listening to him making love to me, just like the wind was making love to the land.

I slid out of bed quietly so as not to wake the kids, flattened out a grease-stained paper bag that had held our chicken dinner, and wrote a poem about the Adirondacks on the back. I tucked it away in the zipper pocket of the map bag.

"I keep hearing myself scream 'NO' when I get turned on."

"Abuse victims often deny what happened to them. What would help you? To have an orgasm?"

He was the doctor, he would know best. "Well ... that might be a good idea," I said hesitatingly. "Where should we do this, on the floor?"

David opened his palm and gestured to the carpet. "Sure."

"Unless you have a nice cozy bed available in your closet?" We both laughed.

"Before we do this, we should have a new contract." The light from the window glanced off David's glasses. He took them off and polished them.

"A new contract." I wondered what he had in mind. "So I can't report you for being sexual with me."

"Oh, I'm not worried about *that*." David waved his hand in the air nonchalantly as if brushing away a fly, "I'd only get my wrist slapped anyway."

"Well, what do you want in the contract?"

"I think you have intimacy issues and I think you should look at me while you touch yourself. The rules are, you look at me, I can touch you to connect with you and you can touch you to connect with you. But you can't touch me. You can take your clothes off, but mine stay on."

"Oh, I get it, so it will appear that you receive no sexual gratification. That way you're safe. We can play with fire, but not get burned."

"Right. But I would be with you in a very powerful way."

David closed the blinds and turned out the light attached to the foot of the examination table. He put the pillow from the examination table on the carpet for my head and covered it with a disposable cloth. He smoothed out the wrinkles and then sat down cross-legged in front of the makeshift bed while he leaned his back against the examination table.

He watched me while I bounced on one leg, taking my underwear off from under my skirt. I kept falling over and grabbing at things so I wouldn't pitch over in a heap. What a klutz. He laughed. Did he want my skirt off as well? Maybe I'd leave it on for that "air of mystery," as Richard would say. *Oh Richard, what would you think of all this?* I lay on the floor in front of David and he placed his hand on my breast so that he would be connected to me.

I felt frozen. "Do you think it would help me if I told you a fantasy about us?"

"Well, fantasy gets you ready for the real thing."

The real thing? Was that sex with him? Did I want sex with him? I desperately wanted to please him, I knew that. I desperately wanted him to love me back. I put my hand under my skirt and he locked eyes with me.

"Because you hear a 'no' in your head, perhaps you should say 'Yes Daddy'. I am your good, loving Daddy." He smiled at me.

He watched my hand moving under my skirt and then stared at me. He rocked back and forth as he sat cross-legged beside me. A vein throbbed in his neck. His breathing was laboured.

"I'm frightened, Daddy."

"Nothing will happen, I'm with you in a very powerful way. I am a good, loving daddy. Say 'Yes Daddy' to me. Look right at me." He fondled my breast.

"Yes Daddy." I breathed faster and faster as David rocked beside me. He was *with* me. I whispered "Yes Daddy" over and over again while our eyes locked together.

I felt like my brain and body were being hotwired to his, we were in such perfect connection. I felt we were bound together in a magical spell. Afterwards he asked me, "How are you feeling now?"

"I love the way you look at me. Were you making love to me in your head?"

David smiled at me so gently. "Yes. I *did* say I would be with you in a very powerful way."

"So, I guess that's what they call a 'mindfuck,' huh? You can fuck my head any day. That's quite some bedside manner."

As we were hugging good-bye I whispered into his ear, "Do I turn you on, David?"

He tilted his head back and smiled at me. "You turn me on incredibly. I fight it constantly."

I laughed and tapped his bum, "Hmm. Sometimes you lose the fight, huh?" I giggled off and on, all the way home.

That night in my office I placed a piece of paper in the pool of light on my desk and began to write about how we had become an eternal, shimmering oneness and how I loved the way he looked at me, with his singing white-hot light. That night I drank nine beers. Again Richard told me I was drinking too much. I knew I was, but I didn't know why. I responded absently, "Oh. Sorry."

Over and over David and I negotiated the contract for self-stimulation sessions. David made my "bed" and laughed with me as I stumbled while undressing. I lay in front of him naked from the waist down and told him fantasies about us while electricity charged from his eyes to mine, binding us together.

I couldn't believe how much it was snowing. David was going to Hamilton the next day for a course he was taking. As I fried pork chops I heard on the radio that even the snowplows were sliding off the roads. I had better leave a note on his car telling him to be careful. Richard hadn't come home from work yet. I hoped he was safe.

With promises of a trip to the candy store, I packed the kids into the car and drove up to David's office, explaining that I had to leave a note for my doctor who was working late. I'd placed my note in a sandwich bag to keep it dry and hooked it under his windshield wiper. I gave his car a good luck pat. I'd die if anything happened to him.

David was furious. He held my note tightly between white fingertips and was stabbing the air with it. "You left a note on my car," he accused. Why was he so mad? Because I loved him? I registered that the note had survived the weather. Good idea, that baggy.

"Yeah, I was worried about the freezing rain," I mumbled.

"I find it annoying." He spat with cruel venom, "*You* are annoying." And then he went ballistic, raising his voice.

"Who needs this shit? Get out of my office! There are lots of therapists out there!" He was shouting at the top of his lungs, his hand punching the air.

Would he hit me? Could Lydia hear? Jesus Christ, it was just a note. What was wrong with him?

He was aiming his fingers at me as he struck the air with the note. I felt like the room was filled with swirling razor blades. I staggered from his office. I was such a bad person. I would try harder so he would love me and not shout.

I was looking down at my hands, playing with my wedding ring. My heart pounded with fear. For the first time ever I would challenge him. "I really hate being shouted at David. It was on my list, remember? I talked to my husband about this and he said that people make mistakes and that I should talk to you."

"You talked to your husband?" David's voice was shrill. "*About us? About what we do?*"

"No, never, it's just that I was obviously really upset when I got home. He asked me what was wrong and I told him you were mad at me. That's all. He said that I should just talk to you and clear it up."

David was smouldering. "Our relationship was never in question. If you're anxious about me in any way, talk to *me* about it. Not other people. Don't talk to your husband about what goes on in here. This is *our* relationship."

"But you hurt me. You said I was 'annoying.'"

"I'm sorry I said that. I was angry. You're not annoying. The note on my car was annoying. There's a difference between you and the behaviour. Our relationship is confined to in here." He gestured widely around the room with his hands. "Not out there. I won't get sexual with you out there." He pointed towards the window. "This, in here, this room is a safe place for sex."

What would Richard say about that? Guilt consumed me.

Weeks and weeks went by. David continued to touch me sexually. I was grateful that he loved me and was treating me kindly. The sessions were full of re-parenting hugs on the floor for "anxiety," goodbye hugs at the door, rape scenes, body scans, rewirings, and lying on the carpet in front of him while he watched. I turned forty-three.

One day I was daydreaming about how attracted I was to him while he was rambling on about this and that. Suddenly, my ears perked up. Oh my god, what was he saying? Did I get that right?

"Pardon?"

"I would certainly find you very attractive outside the office and would enjoy a relationship with you. I would be interested in having a loving sexual relationship with you, but not in this setting."

What? I had better clarify this. He'd asked me before for a relationship outside his office and then said he hadn't asked me. I was going to make him spell this out!

"Are you are asking me to have a relationship with you in your personal life? A relationship where we go out together and see how we get along as a man and a woman? A relationship that does not involve this office? You *personally* would like to have a relationship with me *personally* outside this office?"

"Yes. I would like to have a relationship with you, but not in this setting."

A wild emotion coursed through me. But something was wrong. I felt so upset. Why couldn't I figure this out? "I will have to think about it. I'll let you know. Thanks though."

I was dizzy with confusion. I was madly in love with David, I believed that with all my heart. But was it love? I loved my darling Richard. That felt so different. But then I was married to him. Not that I thought about him much lately. My heart hurt.

Finally, a week later, I was brave enough to approach the subject. "You asked me to have a relationship with you outside this office."

"I never asked you for a relationship outside the office."

Oh, for heaven's sake, this is exactly what he'd done before. "Yes you did, David. You said, last week, very clearly, that you would like to have a relationship with me, but not in this setting."

"When I said 'not this setting,' I meant 'not this life.'"

So he admitted saying it. He corrected part of his lie. "No, you didn't, David, you definitely asked me. That's why I asked you if you meant in your *personal* life."

"Well, it's just not something I can do."

I was devastated and relieved at the same time. It was probably just as well. I really loved Richard. I stood up and gave him a hug. "Easy come, easy go."

He spat, "You can play with it. But I won't play with it."

What did that mean? Play with what? He had that look in his eye that Lynn used to get. I had to get out, fast.

"Gotta go."

He chased me down the hallway. I could feel his ragged breath on my neck. "You can play with it. I won't."

What on earth did he mean? I ran past the waiting room while he charged after me. I burst through the storm door and he finally stopped when it slammed in his face. I turned around and could see his eyes glinting in the bright afternoon sunlight, his breath fogging the glass around his mouth. I flew down the stairs. I had to get away from him. I stood panting by my car. What had I done wrong? What did I have to do to get him to love me? He felt so dangerous. When I got home I ate my lunch in fast gulps. I had stood up to him before when he shouted at me. It didn't go great, but I knew if I were sitting in the waiting room and saw a doctor chasing a patient into the street I would think it was very bizarre. I'd had enough of his anger.

I punched his office number and tersely made a five-minute appointment.

I stood ramrod straight in front of him. "How dare you follow me into the street. All those people in the waiting room saw you chasing me."

"I think you're angry because I rejected you."

"Are you kidding? I'm angry because you're a ... what's the word for a male version of a cock tease? You lead me on and then get angry at me. That's what you do. You do things to turn me on and then punish me because I respond. You flip the flip. You shouted at me. In front of people. Why were you so angry? That I didn't care you'd changed your mind? You know what you are Blackwood? You're a mindfucking bastard."

"Has it come to this? To name-calling? Don't call me names."

"It's not a name. It's who you are. I'll call you a mindfuck if you behave like a mindfuck."

He shouted, "I think you'd better leave now."

"Just what I was planning to do." I turned around at the door. "See you tomorrow." Where did *that* come from?

I didn't remember getting in my car. I felt my ground had been ripped apart by an earthquake and I was gripping the muddy sides of a widening gulf with my fingernails, trying desperately not to fall down into the opening chasm. It felt like he was fracturing my soul and the sea was roaring in. I felt like I was in the center of a volcano with black waves of fear and love swirling around me. I waited with my head on the steering wheel until the noise in my ears subsided.

I finally lifted my head and looked around at the too bright world. I reassured myself that I was indeed back on the surface of the earth. Somehow I remembered that there were things I had to do. I rummaged in my purse for my daily list and checked it. Emma needed a highlighter and we were out of bread. I backed out of my parking spot and headed towards the drugstore.

CHAPTER 8

I
T WAS DINNERTIME AND my son Jamie, his blue eyes wide with
injustice, announced to the table, "I'm ten, you know."
"Yes, I know," I laughed.
"So, I'm growing up without a dog."
"Your mother is allergic to dogs, Jamie." Richard admonished.
"Yeah, but you can get non-allergenic puppies. See?" He put the clas-
sified ads on the table and pointed to a few columns of tiny print.
"No reading at the table," I laughed as I held the paper at arm's
length, trying to focus on the blurry print. Was I so old now that I
needed reading glasses?
"This is serious, Mom. I want a dog. I know you're allergic to like ev-
erything and I wouldn't want you to suffer, but we could have a poodle
mix, something small, like this one here." He tapped the paper.
Emma, Margaret, and Richard all started to talk excitedly. A dog!
The next day I was driving home from a local farm with the cutest
ball of fluff sleeping on a pillow in the back seat. The three kids were
cooing and patting it gently. I named him 'King'."

Life in David's office went on as if nothing had happened, appointments
filled with body scans and rewirings. But he had frightened me and I
decided that I wouldn't hug him anymore. I missed our daily hugs and
touching the landscape of his soul while he held me softly. But I knew
if we got too sexually close, he would punish me somehow. He would
do something to remind me that I was merely a patient to him, even
though I knew I was not. Maybe he did it to remind himself. He would
keep me waiting for my appointment, or he would distance himself by
taking notes, or he would cut my hour in half, or he wouldn't let me
know he couldn't make it and my appointment was cancelled. Then
I would try harder to get him to love me by doing what he wanted.
I would beg for affection. But now I was wise to his game and had

had enough. I kept my distance so I wouldn't get hurt. But, I missed his hugs.

We were winding up another session and for the first time in weeks he held his arms open. He missed our goodbye hugs, too? Should I or shouldn't I? He solved my dilemma by stepping forward and wrapping his arms around me. I melted into him. But then he tensed. He gripped my shoulders. And then he pushed.

He pushed me!

I banged into a chair, regained my balance and ran out of his office, a sob catching in my throat. When I got halfway down the hall, I stopped. He wasn't allowed to *push* me.

I turned on my heel. He looked up from writing in my chart.

"You don't need to push me." My pulse beat wildly. Challenging him was a huge effort. He was my god and could do no wrong. But he had! "Pushing is unacceptable."

"Okay."

"I'll go on my own accord."

"Okay."

"Use your words, you don't need to be physical."

"Okay."

I left his office feeling proud that I'd stood up for myself. I didn't care if I wasn't pleasing him. I would not be pushed. I'd made my point.

The next day he brought up the incident. "I wasn't aware that I had pushed you."

I rolled my eyes. "I'm such a victim, even my therapist abuses me."

"No one has ever said that I'm violent."

"I'll tell you the next time you're pushing me, so you'll know that you are." My sarcasm hung in the air.

The push haunted me for weeks and I felt better keeping my distance. There were no hugs. Again. Finally, after a month of dancing around each other in the office, David broached the subject. "There was no malicious intent in the push. It was just a gesture of communication."

So now he admits it? But I didn't want to fight anymore. I missed our song of songs. Besides, I'd thought more about why he kept punishing me with his distance and aloofness and lies. Once, after a steamy session, he had pulled out a pad of paper from his desk drawer and started taking notes about what I was saying. I watched him write, sitting up straight with his nose in the air, his shoulders stiff as if he were proving he wasn't engaged in what we were talking about. Maybe he was frightened of being loved by me. Or maybe by his loving me. That's why he had to act like an overly professional doctor. "That's okay David, don't worry about it."

That night in my office I pushed my pen firmly into the page and dug out the word "Lies." He'd asked me to have a relationship outside his office and then said he hadn't. Lie. He said he loved me like a child and wasn't sexually involved with me but he got an erection when he held me. Lie. He said I didn't turn him on and then admitted I turned him on incredibly and he had to fight it constantly. Lie. After he said, "Who needs this shit, get out of my office, there are lots of therapists out there," he said our relationship was never in question. Lie. After he got turned on when he taught me foreplay he said it was all *my* energy. Lie. He'd said "I won't get sexual with you" and then said, "this room is a safe place for sex." He told me I was annoying and then said he meant it was the *behaviour* that was annoying. Lies, all lies. And now the latest of lies: he said he didn't push me. Then he said it was a gesture of communication. Lies and more lies.

Two days later I sat nervously in front of him. I was going to challenge him yet again. "You lie to me David. You say one thing and then take it back. Or say you mean something else." I went through the list with him. He seemed to be shrinking in front of me.

His hand jerkily poked at his glasses and he was panting through lips that were stretched across his teeth. Dr. Blackwood did not like being caught in a lie. Or twenty. He said, "I feel smashed. Shattered. Attacked. I feel I have been taken over in my brain."

I was the one being lied to and *he* was the victim? I looked at him with my mouth open. "Taken over in his brain"? A simple sorry and a promise not to do it again would have done the job. At least he didn't shout or hit me.

I felt as if my marriage with Richard was falling apart. I didn't know how he felt, but I felt I was in the Arctic, stumbling through the dark tundra, peering through cold Arctic air for a glimpse of fire, hope, anything light. My relationship with David gave me all that now and it seemed as if Richard was left in the cold. When I thought about leaving the love of my life, fingers of frozen wind iced around my heart. I only wanted it to be a warm summer again for Richard and me. One night I sat at my desk with my pad of paper in front of me and wrote a poem called "Tundra." The next day I read it to David.

"I feel like that David. I am no longer that interested in Richard. It hurts me."

David was hemming and hawing and my mind wandered while I waited for him to make up yet another lie.

And then I heard him say, "...like I was madly in love with you."

I really should pay better attention. I had certainly missed something there. I felt I had better say something and not look a complete dolt. "Oh."

"I talk about my issues with my therapists." He had more than one therapist?

"Oh." What do you say to that? How many therapists does he need? Perhaps one for each leg he doesn't have to stand on.

But what about my marriage?

"I have to stop now." David's voice was hoarse.

I was lying on the examination table and David was standing beside me, his foot resting on the stepstool. It was another body scan.

"Why?" I tried to move his hand, but it wouldn't budge.

"No, I can't do anymore today."

I looked at him. He had deliberately pressed his right knee out as far as it would go, putting the bulge in his blue pants three inches from my face. Fear burst through my skin and my whole body screamed "No, No, NO!" It was supposed to be a body scan. It wasn't supposed to be sexual. I desperately wanted him to stop putting his erection in my face. I stared at it with horrid fascination. It looked softer than the ones in my back. It veered off to the side.

"Yes, I can't do anymore today. This is not a rejection of you."

I could certainly see that.

Afterwards I sat in my car and leaned my head back against the headrest. What was wrong with me? Even after all that work, all those fantasies about him, when I was faced with the real thing, I was terrified. I couldn't respond. There was something wrong with me. I drove home weeping.

Richard stood behind me and put his arms around me while I was stirring a cheese sauce. "Are you okay honey? You seem upset."

"Um, yeah. Yeah, I'm fine sweetheart." I wasn't allowed to talk to Richard anymore about what was going on in Blackwood's office. Something fractured in my soul as I tried to live in two worlds. I placed plates of macaroni and cheese in front of my family and wondered if David would like it.

The next day David tried to make me talk about what had happened. I wished he would just shut up. "It wasn't a rejection of you. If you saw anything or felt anything we should talk about it."

I said, "David, if a man presses an erection against a woman, does he want her to touch it?"

The question hung in the air.

"Yes."

"I wouldn't be able to do that." I started to cry.

"That's okay, fantasy will get you ready for the real thing."

"I should fantasize in my head what happened yesterday but create a new ending? One where I touch your penis and then we make love?"

"It would help you get ready for the real thing. Make it your homework. Fantasize it while you masturbate. Do it every day."

I would follow the doctor's orders. In the ending of my fantasy I would be able to touch him and make love to him.

I would do my homework.

I missed David so much during the Christmas holidays at the cottage. I paced in the snow like a thirsty wolf at the edge of the half-frozen lake. The wind howled across the water and flung broken pieces of ice onto the shore. I watched them shatter over and over again. The shards of ice glinted like razor blades in the moonlight and stabbed the air with the sharp edge of my longing.

I paced and paced on the shore and imagined swallowing the broken lake. I knew how it would feel as it sliced into my soul until I vomited a howl of blood. In that terrible moment, imagining my cry congealing as it was caught between the night and the lake, I understood why wolves howled at the moon. I missed him so badly I could hardly breathe. I told him all this when I got back into the safety of his office.

"You sound like you're ready to have a relationship with me outside the office."

My heart sank. I wasn't going to fall for *that* again. Did he think I was stupid? I was going to be forty-four this summer, a woman of the world! But maybe a relationship outside the office was just what we needed. He wouldn't be conflicted about being a doctor to a patient he was in love with. I'd think about it.

I said, "We can talk about that later."

That summer I went back to Nova Scotia. One night I went for a long walk on the beach with the endless longing refrain of "David David David" travelling through my veins. I listened to the soft windy roar of the open sea and watched the waves swirl over and caress the sand with foam. I took off my clothes and lay down in the frothing white waves, imagining his hand loving me just like the waves did as they washed over me with a quiet caress. He was my god in nature.

David was going away again. This time to Ottawa. He'd be leaving in a few weeks. We both knew that a sexual event would tide us over the separation, and he suggested a flip the flip and a sexual body scan done on the same day. A double-whammy, so to speak.

At the end of the exercises I whispered up at him from the examination table, "You look like you want to kiss me. Do you?"

David jumped back, a damp patch remaining where his hand had been, "NO! No kissing."

That again. He was so conflicted. He loved me like a man, but he had to behave like a doctor. Or was it he was frightened of being loved or of loving? Whatever. I had had enough. I drove home and said over and over, "Enough is enough, enough is enough." I knew I had to do something.

"Lydia? Hi, it's Kathy."

"David's left for the day he went home early. Headache or something."

Yeah, more like penis ache. I put on my calmest voice. "Please tell Dr. Blackwood that our office relationship is over. Tell him thank you very much for all the help, but I won't be coming anymore."

I wondered if Lydia got the pun, or was she as dimwitted as David?

Oh god, what had I done? That night I understood that I was totally in David's power. I drank enough so that my hands would stop shaking and picked up a pen and began to write and write. I wrote how he was a cat and I was a bird with broken wings and couldn't get away. I wrote that I was terrified as he stalked around me, his tail twitching, looking for a good moment to pounce and kill me, to toss me in the air and toy with me as my feathers flew. I felt so helpless. My only recourse was to play dead, to lie very still. I would be safe from him then because he'd sniff the air for other prey. It was a waiting game. I called the poem "Playing Dead."

Something very bad was happening inside my head. I felt like my brain was fraying and I was being trapped in the threads of madness. I sat and drank and wrote. I couldn't stop myself; escaping reality and falling into madness was so seductive.

The next poem I wrote was about the hiss of spinning chaos beckoning to me like a snake in the Garden of Eden. There was a temptation to eat the fruit of madness, to become one with it, to have it enter me. That would be a sweet surrender, a narcotic to give me peace of mind. The chaos was a transparent pool of watery insanity. It took every ounce of my spirit to not dive in. I wrote how I planted my feet into the forest floor of damp oblivion so that I would be held safely in the dark earth. I would not succumb to the temptation. I called the poem "Temptation."

I drank and drank and had to write more. I wrote how the inner edge of madness looked like a galaxy turned inside out. How white spinning stars churned with a loud, never ending explosion, yet there was no sound at all except for the steady beat of an ancient heart, pulling and pushing and pulling away from the slow, suffocating wall of endless spinning air. I wrote how it created a vacuum of nothingness that kept trying to suck me in.

I wrote how I needed something to keep me safe from the imploding black hole of my universe. Where could I go for help? I felt as if my fingers were scraping and clawing into nothing while I was being sucked into the vortex of madness. I needed David so badly to hold me and keep me away from the madness. The last line of the poem was "Where are you?" I called this poem "Help."

I picked up the telephone and left a message on his office voice mail. "Oh, hi David, it's me, Kathy. I'm so sorry I asked Lydia to tell you our relationship was over. Of course it isn't. I'll see you tomorrow."

"There," I whispered, "it's okay, Kathy, everything's okay." *Kathy?*

Again! I hadn't thought of myself as Kathy in a long time. I was Sky. What was happening to me? Cold shivers went down my spine. I snuck into bed and got as close as I could to Richard without touching him.

He rolled towards me, "God, you're cold, come here."

My world was splintering. I went into his arms and fell asleep knowing that I had to get my relationship with David out of that damn office.

CHAPTER 9

DAVID WAS SMILING AS he talked about his upcoming trip to Ottawa. Did he want me to come? He shrugged, a small grin on his face. He did? A trip? Ottawa! He told me where he'd be staying! The name of his conference! Hooray! Finally we'd get out of his grubby office with its ridiculous contracts. He would be free to love me without the restrictions of being my doctor. And if his erratic behaviour was because he was frightened of loving me or being loved, I would be patient. But not his "patient."

I made some excuses to Richard about why I needed to go to Ottawa and was flabbergasted by how easy it was to trick him. Was he fooled? What was happening to our marriage? Did he know about me and David? Oh god, I hoped not. The thought of hurting my darling Richard, the love of my life, broke my heart. Why did I have to be with David? It felt as if my head was splitting apart.

As the miles ticked by on the highway to Ottawa, I rehearsed out loud all the great lines I would say to David. I had to be so smart. I needed him to love me back.

I found a downtown hotel, hefted my bags out of the trunk, and booked myself in. After I unpacked, I got out the love poem I had written for him and put it in a hotel envelope I found in the desk drawer. I wondered if he'd notice where I was staying.

How to get the poem to David? I looked at an Ottawa map, got my bearings, and slowly found my way over to his hotel, searching out street names and matching them to my map. About a minute later I saw it, the Minto. Geez, I was staying less than a block away. Silly me.

I struggled with the huge glass doors, but finally got inside, the envelope only slightly creased. I tried to flatten out the crumpled paper on the sparkling reception desk while a receptionist watched me, amused. My hands were grimy from the door and now the crumples had smudge marks. This was not going well.

I searched the hotel's schedule board and found the room number of his conference. I trotted down the hall, entered an enormous foyer and faced two huge white doors. Things were looking up: I knew where he was. Behind those big white doors.

The very empty foyer reminded me of Versailles, what with the flowered carpet and curlicued white chairs lined neatly along a wall. A bellhop strode up to me on feet that barely whispered on the carpet. I felt like an out of place bag lady, an interloper in foreign territory. But he was looking at me earnestly, curiosity crinkling the skin around his eyes.

"Can I help you with anything, ma'am?"

Ma'am? Surely I wasn't a ma'am. Not yet. I showed him the less than pristine envelope and said, "I would like this to be delivered to David Blackwood. He's behind those white doors."

"Certainly ma'am."

Jesus, when did "ma'am" happen to me?

He took the envelope, opened the doors and strode in. Just like that I had accomplished my goal of the day. David would know I was here. I sat in one of the French provincial chairs facing the room and waited for the white doors to open. I was so excited. As I perched in the huge chair I felt like a six-year-old, swinging my feet back and forth, unable to reach the carpet.

Finally the doors swung wide and he burst through, backlit like an angel. My heart soared. He was wearing the blue sweatshirt I had given him for Christmas. He loved me. Oh dear, I should have gotten him the extra large. As he got closer I could see his mouth was a deep gash carved across his face and the glare from his eyes stabbed at me with anger.

"What are you doing here? You shouldn't have come here. I am going to call hotel security."

Wait a sec. He'd told me he was going to be here. Did I get something wrong? And now he was striding away. I had to run to keep up. How embarrassing.

"David, don't be mad." I felt like hitting him. My fist curled into a tight little ball. He reminded me of my older brother. "David, don't be mad at me. I thought you asked me to come."

"I can't ask you to my room. I'm sharing it with someone else. I don't know where we can go to talk."

"Here, we can talk right here." I pointed to a little alcove with a telephone and a love seat.

We parked on the edges of the small couch, deliberately not touching, and I watched his hands turn glacier white as they strangled a stack of loose papers.

"Why are you so angry at me? I was sure you wanted me to come."

"I was kidding. We have an office-based relationship. It takes two to dance. Our relationship belongs in my office, not in life."

I should have known. "I always felt like you were dancing with me, David. Things happen in that office that should only happen in life."

His anger was a cold winter gale. "Maybe so. Maybe so."

Suddenly he leapt off the sofa and sprang towards the elevator. My jaw dropped. My heart pounded in my ears and my head spun chaotically. Frustration and anger, confusion and doubt, certainty and love, swept over me. I thought I was going to faint.

The elevator opened and he wedged himself into the crowd. He whipped his head around and glowered at me as the steel doors slid together.

I shouted across the room before they closed, "You have to face yourself David Blackwood. You have to face yourself."

I ran to the elevator but the doors whapped shut, leaving me standing in the lobby, my words echoing loudly, my face a wobbly reflection in the buffed metal. What a fiasco. People were looking at me. I didn't care. I stumbled back to my hotel, not seeing where I was going.

I looked out of my hotel bedroom at the Ottawa River looping around a curve while I went around my own personal bend. I didn't know how I had gotten back to the room, but I knew I had to keep looking at the river. I knew I had to love it as it curled around the landscape and I imagined it was curling around my soul just as David had done. I watched the river flow lazily until after night fell and then slowly ate a sandwich I had brought from home. I cracked open a beer and felt my nerves settle down as I lost myself in a good mystery book.

The sharp ring of the phone made me jump. Beer went everywhere. Should I answer? What if it was David?

"Hello?"

"I have a message for you from David Blackwood. He wanted me to read it to you."

Read it? Wasn't there a message machine with a flashing light on the phone? Yes, there it was, a little green square with "Messages" written under it. What a coward: he didn't want to call and risk talking to me.

"Okay, go ahead."

The receptionist began to read. "If you contact me, I will call hotel security. Do not try to meet me in any way. I am not available to you. I will see you only in Toronto." She stopped reading, her voice garbled with embarrassment. My heart went out to her.

"Oh, poor you for having to read me a message like that. Never mind. He and I will work it out."

I sat down and chewed my lip while I composed a letter to David. I outlined my three basic requirements for a relationship. One was to never walk away and leave the other person stranded in the middle of a discussion. Two was to be honest; I knew he'd asked me to Ottawa. And three was to never threaten and play hardball. I remembered how he had pushed me and wrote that I could play hardball as well and threaten him with calling the police. I walked calmly over to his hotel and delivered it to his front desk.

The next morning he wrote me back just the sweetest apology with explanations for his rude behaviour. He was involved here. I had surprised him. The issue had become polarized. But he couldn't see me. He was sorry but he couldn't make plans: his mother was sick; he might have to leave Ottawa quickly. I raced through the words frantically until I got to the end. Ah ha! He suggested we discuss a future kind of relationship at my next appointment.

All was not lost. He did love me. He wanted to move the relationship out of the office.

I flung my belongings into my suitcase. I had to get out before I had to pay for another day. I went down to the front desk and begged to be released from my booking. I recognized the voice of the nice girl behind the counter as the one who had read me the ghastly message.

"No problem. It's still before eleven. Did everything work out okay?"

"Yes, everything's perfect!"

I drove back to Toronto with the promise of a connection with David fuelling me all the way. Yes, this would be our very last appointment. He loved me, sure he did. That's why he said we would have a relationship outside his office. He wrote it down in his beautiful lovely letter.

Other drivers looked at me oddly as I whizzed past, happily spewing out line after line as I rehearsed what I would say during my last therapy session with David, laughing and laughing as the miles flew by.

While David was away at his conference I tried to occupy myself so I wouldn't miss him so much. One windy night I sat in Nathan Philips Square and imagined that the wind was like water cascading around me, caressing me like David's hands. I imagined that the arrow of the Archer, the rounded abstract sculpture by Moore in the center of the square, was swimming in the wind up my skirt, touching me where I ached for him.

I pulled out an old shopping list from my purse and wrote on the back "The Archer." Hope, fear, and homesickness for him all surfaced for air inside my heart, with each emotion pushing the other down in a teeter-totter of drowning confusion. Waiting for him to come home was hell.

Finally the date of my last appointment arrived and I drove to his office carefully. I nervously sat in front of him, my feet tightly hooked around each chair leg. I felt I was blathering.

"I feel better, David."

He looked at me with pleasure.

"I don't feel under the ice," I said. "The lake is no longer frozen." I looked at him to see if he was getting my references to poems that I had written to him. I couldn't tell. He was just staring at me. "I feel confident in myself. That's why I could actually go to Ottawa to see you. I have confidence in myself. I want to thank you for holding me while I spun in your arms."

"That's a therapist's job. I'm glad you are cured. I think you've turned a lot of your traumatic memories into normal memories."

It was time for me to bite the bullet and get down to what was going to happen next. "So…" My heart was beating hard in my chest. Why was I so frightened? "You mentioned in your letter that we could get together."

"Yes, I thought we could go out for a drink or a meal to catch up and see what we thought of each other. Would you like that?"

And finally get rid of his conflict? Of course I would. My heart was doing crazy somersaults. Was this from excitement?

"Sure." I felt understatement was best. I added a shrug so I looked blasé.

"The College has rules about how long doctors have to wait before we see our patients socially. It's six months."

"Six MONTHS?"

He raised his eyebrows at my outburst.

"But David, I'll miss you too much. I won't last."

I had been seeing him almost daily for two and a half years and was absolutely dependent upon him. He was in my head. I only existed as a human being in relationship to him. I knew the separation would be torment.

"Well, call me if you need to. But it's really better if we wait."

"Where should I call? Here at the office?"

"No, at home."

"What about your wife?"

"Don't worry about that."

His wife was a "that"?

"But we won't see each other until the fall."

"Okay," I sighed.

We stood up for our final hug in his office. As I held him I could hear his heart beating softly in his chest. I stroked his back, trying to memorize how he felt so I wouldn't forget him over what was going to be a very long summer.

For the last time I whispered in his ear, "I love you."

I waited for him to say "I love you" back as he sometimes did, but I could see his pretty pink lips clamped shut in a determined effort to say nothing.

Oh, for Christ's sake.

That night I scurried through my mind for a good-bye gift idea. I wanted to reimburse him for the many very short visits where he'd hug me so I could get through another day. Surely he hadn't billed OHIP for giving and getting hugs.

I remembered the day we'd been talking about what he ate for lunch and he'd answered a sandwich. I'd asked him why he didn't bring a plateful of food from home and nuke it in the microwave. That's what Richard did with the plates of food I prepared for him. David had said that there wasn't a microwave in the office and he doubted there'd ever be one. What a great idea. I'd get one from Canadian Tire!

I typed him an adoring good-bye letter about how helpful he had been in curing me. It was full of symbolism and innuendo, praise and love for him.

And then I wrote two poems. David fancied himself a sculptor and my first poem was about how he saw that my potential to be a beautiful woman was trapped in a block of frozen rock. I wrote how his warm hands had caressed and melted the hard sharp corners of the rock because he had to reach the soft curves of the beautiful woman. Every now and then a crystal would nick the skin on his roaming hands and his hot blood would hiss and foam pink on my icy surface. And sometimes his hands hurt with my ache of frozen numbness, but because he loved me and had to reach me, he never stopped stroking his block of frozen rock. One day the ice was completely gone and the beautiful woman was freed. I could move. And the very first thing I did was reach for him.

The next poem I wrote for him was about the pain of separating. It was about how I could hear the sound of flesh ripping, the sinew and bone of the two us being torn apart at the chest as we slowly unwrapped our arms and stepped away. I described how the air between us filled up with blood as we moved back from each other. I was swimming in this blood and was desperate with thirst for a taste of our air. I hated the taste of the bloody good-bye. I wondered if he'd remember the cave poem about the taste of blood.

I put the letter and two poems together and stuffed them inside the good-bye card I had bought. I wrote in the card, "For all the times you saw me and didn't bill OHIP, Love Kathy." *Kathy.* That's who I was when I was with him. I ran my tongue under the sticky edge and smoothed it shut. I wrote "David" across the front in big bold letters.

A few days after delivering the microwave I got a thank you card from everyone in his office, not just him. I was devastated. On the front was a puppy and some butterflies on a pastel background. Was I three years old? I could tell that Lydia, not David, had picked it out in a hurry from the local drugstore. My feelings were hurt, even before

I opened the card up. The microwave was for him, not for Lydia and Dr. Charles. I read the thank you with the three signatures, ripped the card up, and flung the offensive pieces into the garbage.

CHAPTER 10

IT WAS GOING TO be a long wait before I could see David socially. I dragged myself to my summer cottage. No matter what I was doing I thought about David. Swimming, walking, sailing, playing tennis, shopping, cooking, everything I did was under the dark cloud of missing him. It felt like it was smothering my skull. Were the kids safe? I made great effort to watch them carefully through the fog of David, David, David. Did Richard know? I tried hard to connect to my husband, even though I felt like a radio-controlled robot with David holding the controls.

I also kept thinking about guns.

One day, after the sun had set and night was falling on the lake, I decided to go out in the canoe. To me the lake became the pain of missing David and the canoe seemed to glide through the steely blue numbness of the ache. The gray, black and blue swirls on the water looked like gunmetal bruises.

The absence of his touch felt like the hollow barrel of a cannon pressed against the skin over my heart. As I paddled across the lake I could feel it blasting a circle with jagged edges of torn flesh. I felt this was where our goodbye had randomly exploded, right in the middle of my chest. I placed the paddle over the gunwales and pressed my hand over my heart. This was where it hurt the most. Right where his hand wasn't. I knew then that absence was a loose cannon, that nothingness could be very violent.

A hole was exploding inside me and I had to hug myself to prevent bits of my flesh being blasted all over the lake.

I dragged the kids to Toronto for a weekend. To avoid the intense summer heat I took my curly-haired non-allergenic puppy for a walk very early one Saturday morning and headed over to a local community centre where I knew David took karate. On my way I ran into my neighbour Marion. She and I had chatted in the street and I loved her sense of humour and gentle manner. When she leaned over to pat King, his little tail whipped back and forth like a metronome and he rubbed himself against her. I knew she was a kind person, right then and there.

"Where are you off to?" she asked, straightening up.

"Oh, just on a walk with the pup." To see the doctor who rewired me I added mentally. What would Marion think?

I tugged on King's leash and hurried off. If I were really lucky I would catch a glimpse of David after his Saturday class. As I rounded a corner, a far away tiny version of David walked towards me. What luck! Oh, how I loved him. I saw his small blue station wagon parked about halfway along the block and quickened my pace. I wanted to get there before he drove away without seeing me and saying hello.

I felt light-headed and wondered if I would disappear as I hurried towards him under the canopy of green leaves. My heart floated in my mouth. My stomach had lurched over and was squeezing my boiled egg and toast. I counselled myself to be normal, be normal.

"Hi David, how are you? It's nice to see you."

I could hardly see straight. It was like I was here but not here. I watched myself wave happily at him.

He was pissed off. "What are you doing here?"

He took out his key and angrily jabbed it into his door lock. Metal scraped against my eardrum. He didn't look at me. I saw the light shining on his chestnut hair as he got into his car. I wanted to touch it. Why wasn't he happy to see me?

"Oh, I'm just walking my dog before it gets too hot. Imagine bumping into you like this. I miss you David."

I felt dizzy. Why wouldn't he look at me?

"I don't miss you." He pulled his leg into his car, slammed the door, and clenched the wheel. I could see his alabaster knuckles through the windshield.

I watched in disbelief as he thrust the key into the ignition, snapped it on, and drove off without a single look, his car sputtering as a few drops of something clear dripped out of its exhaust.

"Bye…" Again I watched myself wave, this time only half-heartedly.

I looked down to see what had dripped out of his exhaust pipe. Was it oil? Gas? Water? I couldn't tell. I looked up as his car disappeared around the corner. And all this from a man who said he would never hurt me. I had believed him.

Trust in the relationship. That's what he had said.

Why was he so angry? Just a few weeks before we had been embracing in his office. Now it was as if he had erupted like a volcano and the molten lava of his anger was spewing everywhere. It had flowed across my skin like a burning river and hardened around the memory of us embracing. His anger had solidified around our entwined bodies, petrifying us in rock. If an archeologist found us like this, what would he make of it? The doctor got angry because I loved him? Or was it because he loved me? Who was petrified, me or him? I chewed at the double entendre.

I lugged myself and my little dog home trying to justify David's behaviour. It was all the same, really. It was just like in his office. Whenever he thought he loved me, he had to be cruel to me. So, he was still doing that. He was frightened of loving a woman. My heart went out to him. He was forgiven. I would persevere. I would never hurt him.

That night I sat in my office and wrote "After Lava."

I hauled the kids back to the cottage where I felt David everywhere in the landscape. One morning I went out for a paddle just as the sun was coming up. Mist swirled around me and it felt as if my canoe was gliding and sliding through the soft water of his soul. Oh god I missed him. Finally the summer ended, leaving just three months left to go before we could date.

Emma was now in high school, trekking across town with Richard on his way to work. Margaret had grown unbelievably, and at twelve was five inches taller than I, which made her easy to spot if I were picking her up from an event. And Jamie, now nine, was getting his gear ready for the fall hockey season. Through all the events of my daily life, driving here and there, making dinner for the kids, making love with Richard, I only thought about David. I felt I no longer existed. I had come to be "us."

Being apart from him created a frightening gap in my mind and I filled that gap by obsessively putting myself in places where he might be. I had to see him to stay alive. He loved me, didn't he? That's why he had touched me all over my body, because he loved me.

I walked down roads where he might be riding his bike home from work. I waited on street corners. I peered over fences. Finally, one day I saw him gliding down a hill. He looked like a warrior on a golden steed. My heart rejoiced. Although I called his name, he didn't answer me back. Was he deaf?

That night I called him from a pay phone in a grocery store because I wanted some privacy from my family. "Hi David, how are you?" I could hear a party going on.

"Who's this?"

As if he didn't know. He was the one who had told me he loved my voice. "It's Kathy."

He was guarded. "Oh. Hi."

I couldn't read his mood. The store's doors scraped open. So much for privacy.

"What's up?"

"Not a lot, how about with you?"

"Ah, my pond has an algae bloom. You're the biology guy, how do I fix that?"

"Remember when I told you to do your homework to get you ready for the real thing?"

"Sure I do." I had followed the doctor's orders every day.

"Yeah, well you can stop doing that. You don't need to do it anymore. There are a lot of people here. I should go."

"I saw you on your bike today. My heart just leapt. I just loved seeing you." A trolley wheeled past me, its wheels squeaking.

"Are you still doing that?"

What did he mean? Still doing what?

"Okay, I'll let you go."

What had just happened?

Of course he loved me. That's why he told me to stop doing my homework: this *was* the real thing. We'd had a very beautiful intimate relationship. A blizzard of pain obliterated my heart. I missed him so much. I went into the store and bought eggs.

I was driving along Gray Road #2 on the way to Meaford to visit a friend, muttering away to myself about David, when suddenly I saw in my peripheral vision the silhouette of two trees leaning against the horizon. They were so close together that their trunks and bare

branches had wound around each other, looking like two lovers diving into the earth, waving their legs joyfully in the sky. They were just
like David and me.

I stopped the car and threw it into reverse. The wheels scrunched on
the gravel shoulder of the highway as I backed up, the engine whining
in protest. The car careened wildly as I tried to keep it in a straight
line. Finally I lurched to a stop a few inches from the ditch opposite
the two trees.

I looked at the trees and wondered if I could capture with my camera
the essence of what I saw. I remembered my first rewiring and how
the moment had burned through my retina and was now projected
on my skull. No camera would be fast enough to capture that instant
when spirit, flesh and bone flew around us and disappeared. Could I
capture this?

That night I looked at the photographs I had taken on my computer;
the trees really did look like lovers diving headfirst into the earth. I
wrote a poem about how the land around the trees waved and pulsed
with the music of their roots kissing. I called it "Trees." I directed
David to look closely where their legs married, because it was there
he would see Aphrodite dancing to the soft beat of the land, her rising
pleasure leaning into the song of songs, her hips ripe with open tension.
Waiting was driving me crazy.

But there was something wrong with me, I knew it. Even though he'd
told me to stop doing my homework, to stop masturbating while I
fantasized a new ending to that day when he'd put his penis in my face,
I couldn't stop. I had to do it. Daily. Was I a nympho? How embarrassing. Maybe this happened to forty-four year old women.

Plus, I kept talking out loud in my car. I was rehearsing all the things
I had said to David and all the things I was going to say. It didn't really bother me; it was sort of fun. I made him laugh in these fantastic
daydreams. I was so hilarious. But I knew other drivers were looking
at me. That would shut me up for a bit, but then yak yak yak, I'd be
at it again, laughing away.

And I was driving around his block. I drove past his house at least
once a day. That didn't bother me either. In fact, as I drove around
burbling gaily to him I felt better. It sort of calmed me down. For a
second or two. I never did it so he could see me. Imagine how em-

barrassed I'd be if he saw me talking to myself as I drove in front of his house, laughing like a mad woman. But I couldn't stop myself. I decided I had better find a new therapist. I knew I was sort of nuts. I was worried about it. I couldn't be like my mother. Would I ever work again? I didn't want to turn into a bag lady, pushing a shopping cart, shouting at people.

How long had I been out of control? I tried to remember when I had started rehearsing what I was going to say to him. It was pretty soon after the first time he stroked my breast. Years ago. I was getting worse. I needed help. I knew it.

A few weeks later I was driving around David's house and saw a moving van. His wife was moving out. My heart ached for the pain of his marriage breakdown and then pulsed with fear. He told me he'd leave her for me. Did I want that? I couldn't leave Richard. He was my one true love. So who was David?

I thought about him in his empty house. His pain seemed to be inside me and I tried to comfort myself by holding a shell from my beach to my ear. The gentle echo of the ocean calmed my mind and I knew I had to give the shell to David. I wanted him to hold it to his ear and have a blanket of quiet waves wash over him so he could rest. I wrote a poem for him called "Shellshock."

Later that night I put "Trees," "Shellshock," and the shell into a pretty gift bag and drove over to his neighbourhood. I did a full circle of his block and saw his house was in darkness. I skulked up his path and hung the gift bag from his doorknob.

But where was David? I drove up and down dark streets looking for his blue car. My heart thumped every time I saw one. I wanted to call him and started rehearsing out loud what I would say. Soon I was speaking at a pretty high decibel.

I drove and drove. Why wasn't he with me? I needed to console him. I was fantasizing that I was with him. And then I was shouting at the top of my lungs. *Where are you? Where are you?*

I stopped at a red light and took a breath. *Oh god*, I despaired, *I am so nuts.*

The next day I called a female therapist, a doctor a friend had told me about. I needed help. Fast. I had to be normal for my first date with David and there was something really wrong with my head. It seemed to be hissing his name at me. The only thing in my skull was David, David, David.

I felt frightened. All the time. When I rubbed my arms to calm myself down I couldn't feel them.

CHAPTER 11

THE SUN SHONE THROUGH the sliding glass doors and danced around the room. It filtered through little glass objects placed on the glass table in front of me, leaving rainbow prisms on the walls. The smell of coffee and distant cigarette smoke floated in the air as I fiddled with the threads on the arm of the deep couch. I liked the look of my new therapist, Shirley Stewart.

The dog was another matter. It was a tiny Chihuahua that kept shaking. Chihuahuas had fur, not hair like my puppy, and I was worried I would be allergic to it. I checked my lungs for wheezing. Nothing. A miracle, what with the smells, the cigarette smoke, and the wool carpet. "I'm allergic to dogs."

"Lots of people are."

What to do? Usually when I told people I was allergic to their pets they jumped up and apologetically removed them. Except of course for my parents when as a small child I was strangled with asthma. Shirley didn't budge. I looked at her and waited.

With a wave of her much-ringed fingers, she took a blanket and haphazardly tossed it over the poor little thing. It had curled up beside me and was vibrating against my leg. What was wrong with it? Even though there was only a wall of glass between the office and winter, the room was warm. I wanted to pat the little dog but knew if I did I'd be covered in hives.

The dog stayed. And so did I.

Shirley was asking about my drinking. "How much do you drink?"

"About three beers a day."

"So, you drink about six beers a day."

I looked at her in astonishment.

"Everybody lies about that." And then a deep throated laugh.

"Oh." Yes, I thought, I was going to like this woman. She seemed a bit of a bully, sort of loud and domineering, but Shirley was kind to her dog.

"This is *way* more than social drinking." Shirley wailed out the "way" into two syllables to drive her point home. "You have a problem. How long have you been drinking this much?"

"Ever since I could," I laughed. I thought it was funny. Shirley didn't.

"Right." She slapped some words down into the file on her knee. A painted toenail escaped through a hole in her nylons. She grilled me about my childhood, my marriage, my friends, my health, my past therapy. She scrawled my answers so hard that I could hear the pen scrape through the paper fibers. Shirley did not fool around.

"I can't give you therapy. It's too complicated for a regular doctor like me. Abuse. Alcohol. An emotional affair with your doctor. I deal with women in transition. I'm going to refer you to a psychiatrist."

My heart plummeted. I couldn't wait six months to get help. I was seeing David in two. My skin was numb. I talked out loud all the time. Plus I was now driving around his house more and more. It all had to stop.

"No, I'm fine. I've already had two years of therapy. I *am* a woman in transition. I don't need a psychiatrist."

As I said this the room changed shape and my words echoed in a far off land.

"I'm fine. I'll stop drinking."

"Oh yeah? When?"

"Today."

"After drinking hard for years and years, you're telling me you're going to stop drinking? Today?"

"I need therapy, and if that's the deal, I'll stop."

"If you do, then you can see me. At least that'll get rid of one problem." She flung a few more words into my file.

"I'll see you next week, same time. In the meantime, stop drinking and work on your boundaries."

Boundaries? What was this? Now I had to draw maps? No, that was borders. Out of bounds? Like the ball at a baseball game?

"What do you mean? Like maps? Or like out of bounds?"

"Very funny. You have no boundaries. You let people come in to your life that shouldn't come in. You are like a sponge. Protect yourself.

Put up some walls."

"Oh. I don't understand at all. I've never heard the word 'boundaries' applied to people."

Shirley looked at me as if I had the IQ of a shag carpet. "Imagine there is a plate of metal between you and others, that you're living in a steel tube."

"Oh, like— "

Shirley forged on, "Don't let others in unless you want them to come in. Invite them in only after you decide you like them. Assess them. Tighten up your boundaries."

I got into my car with Shirley's words ringing in my ears. She made sense. I would stop drinking and I would think about boundaries. About deciding who I liked. I liked everybody. Maybe I shouldn't.

I was glad I'd told Shirley it was just an emotional affair with David. If I had told her it was sexual Shirley would undoubtedly report him. Would she ever. That was the last thing I wanted her to do. I would protect David with all my heart.

That Shirley was a battleship.

Six months of waiting to see David were finally up. And the two months of therapy with Shirley had done what? Not much. I drove around his house several times while I rehearsed what I was going to say on the phone. My lines had to be perfect. The problem with rehearsing was the unpredictable nature of the other person's response. So I planned ahead. I made four backup speeches.

I named my car "The Chat Room."

I practiced each reply at full volume. "Hello, David, it's Kathy, would you like to get together? Six months is up." "Ah no, but maybe in a few weeks." "Okay David, talk to you later." "Hello David, it's Kathy, would you like to get together? Six months is up." "Oh sure, let's meet at 6:30." "That's great, see you there." "Hello David…" And so on. Finally I was ready for anything. I called.

"Hello David, it's Kathy. Would you like to get together?"

"So, six months is up. Sure, let's go for coffee."

Coffee? My heart froze. I hadn't rehearsed a coffee answer. Dinner, lunch, a movie, a drink, those I had down pat. He knew I didn't drink coffee. It gave my heart palpitations. Why would he suggest coffee? So I'd say no? Get together for coffee? Shit.

"Sure, coffee sounds fine."

We made plans and met the next weekend at a local café. I sipped my mint tea and watched as he stirred four packets of sugar into his froth-filled cup.

"Don't hold back on my account," I said, looking at the discarded wrappers. He didn't laugh.

David stirred the concoction and lifted the foam-covered teaspoon to his lips. Slowly his pink tongue circled the rim of the spoon as his eyes held mine. I watched, mesmerized. I could hardly breathe as panic consumed me. Was he coming on to me? What does one say exactly in this situation? His tongue caressed the base of the handle. I began to babble.

I blathered on about karate and pets, kids and holidays, whatever I could think of. This date wasn't going like a house on fire. Noises bounced off the cement and glass décor and clamored inside my skull. A major headache was brewing behind my eyebrows.

Finally he finished smacking his lips over the cappuccino. As I stood up to leave, my chair legs scraped metallically against the ceramic tiles. I grit my teeth. David clanged some change onto the metal tabletop as he strode ahead of me. He pushed through the door, letting the thick glass shut in my face. I couldn't believe it! Richard would never go through a door first; he would always hold it open for me.

When we were outside the café, awkwardly saying goodbye, he said, "If you want to, we could get together on an occasional basis."

If I wanted to? I was in love with him. I had to see him. "That would be great."

I drove home with "on an occasional basis" reverberating in my memory. What did it mean? The sun's glare bounced off everything I looked at, and I thought I could actually see the atoms in the air vibrating in the sunshine. I waited at a stoplight, sensing a flicker of knowledge sputtering in a dark niche of my mind. The thought suddenly ignited: maybe he didn't love me. A black wave of pain quickly washed the flicker out. Of course he did.

I knew he loved me and had to see me, that's why he kept driving along my running route. He looked so cute in his little blue car. Every time I saw him my heart raced and my stomach flipped over. It was uncanny, how I could see him almost every day in his blue car yet not see him.

God was throwing us together. It was fate. That was it. Fate. We were meant to be together.

Blue cars were a good omen.

And so The Blue Car Game began. If I saw a blue car, it meant he loved me. If I didn't see one, he didn't love me. I started looking for blue cars everywhere. If I saw a black car, he hated me. But if I saw three blue cars in a row after seeing one black car, well, that meant he loved me after all. It was a perfect game that I always won. If I wasn't winning, I'd change the rules so I would.

Cars of different colours took on symbolic meanings. If I saw a combination of a blue car and a red car, that meant he wanted to have sex with me. A yellow car meant he was happy to be near me. Purple cars were for the deep passion he felt for me. Brown cars were negative and needed two blue cars to correct.

And an orange car? Man oh man, orange cars were *king*. One single orange car would counteract a black car. One orange car meant he would call me. One orange car meant we would marry and live happily ever after. This frightened me, but then again how many orange cars were there in the whole country? Three? The risk was small.

So I looked for orange cars on the highway as I drove across the country to Nova Scotia. While I drove up north to Muskoka. While I drove around his house, now up to thirty times a day. While I was waiting for the one orange car in the world, I would say to myself, "If the third car along is a blue car, then he loves me." I passed the time on the roads counting cars and wishing on them, over and over and over.

If I woke up in the middle of the night I would peer through my vertical blinds, looking for a blue car. Of course he loved me. Of course he did. And voila! There'd be a blue car. I would sit in restaurants distractedly looking out the window, searching in the passing stream of cars for a blue one. There, see, he loved me. As I approached an intersection I would think, "If there are two blue cars at the corner then he loves me." And if there weren't, then I'd simply change the rules.

I always won the game. He loved me.

I was standing on the sidewalk outside my house with my neighbour and now friend, Marion. We'd exchanged confidences over a few lunches and I had told her about David and how I felt about him. We were laughing at the absurdity of being in love with a doctor as we stood on the street and now I was explaining all the ins and outs of The Blue Car Game. I pointed to the corner of the street because I had to show her how it worked.

"See, there's a blue car. That means he loves me. Now I'm going to turn around, wait a minute, and ask the universe if he loves me. When I look back at the corner, I'll bet you there'll be a blue car. The universe will answer 'yes.'" I turned around, mumbled under my breath, "if he loves me I'll see a blue car," and turned back. The tail end of a blue car whizzed past.

"See? It's fate Marion. I always see a blue car when I need to see one. And that's because he loves me."

Marion looked skeptically at me. "You really want to believe this, don't you?"

That night I got into bed the same time as Richard, but before I lay down, I climbed on the bed on my knees and pulled down a slat of the blind on the window behind the bed. I wanted to see one last blue car for the day.

Richard propped himself up on one elbow, laughing at me. "What are you doing, Sky? Praying?"

"Just seeing if my car lights are out."

I was reporting to Shirley on my first date with David. "I started to panic when he licked his spoon really slowly. It took him a long time to get all the foam off, his tongue just kept going around and over the spoon. What does it mean when a guy does that? I mean, I just collapsed and started to babble. What do you say?"

The Bully leaned back and grinned. "You say..." and she paused for effect, "*Lucky spoon.*"

We both roared with laughter.

I wanted Shirley to think I was merely a woman in transition. I didn't want her to know I was off-the-rails nuts. But I knew I was.

"I'm not obsessing about David as much as I used to. I seem to be calmer. But I'm doing this thing with blue cars."

"Blue cars." Shirley's pen dug into her chart.

"Yes, I seem to be looking for them. A lot." I wasn't going to tell her it was a game with rules that ran all day and all night. That the minute I left her office I would be looking for a blue car on the street so I would know that he loved me.

"Do you count them? I had one patient who counted green cars. I told her to focus on her life. And I'm telling you to focus on your life. Not on blue cars." She looked at me sternly over her glasses.

Yeah, right. I decided to leave the blue car situation alone for the time being and went on to something else that was really bothering me.

"I have a pain in my heart. Here." I pointed to my chest.

Shirley jerked up straight, her polyester blouse straining against the numerous rolls around her torso. I could see the white stitching stretching at the seams. Shirley had put her feet on the floor and was leaning towards me. I hadn't seen her move so much in months.

Shirley was alarmed. Urgency shook her voice. "What do you mean? How long has this been going on? When was your last medical check-up?"

Shirley didn't understand.

"No, no, no, it's not physical pain, it's emotional pain. It hurts my heart. Here." I banged on my chest. Shirley winced.

I reassured her. "It's just emotional pain. It's not going to kill me."

Air whooshed out of Shirley's lungs as she sat back in her chair. "Okay. As I said before, focus on your life."

"I'm not sure he really wants to see me again."

"Why not? It sounds as if your date went well."

"He said, 'occasionally.' We'd get together 'on an occasional basis.'" I choked on the words.

Shirley caught herself before her eyes rolled totally back into her head. "Why would you want to be with someone who doesn't want to be with you? Your husband loves you. Resolve the issues in your marriage."

"My husband doesn't love me."

"Yes he does. He loves you in his way. It may not be the way you want him to love you, but he does love you."

I decided not to argue. Shirley would win.

CHAPTER 12

I WAITED AND WAITED for David to call. The silence of the phone was deafening. It was important that *he* call *me*, because I didn't want to be with someone who didn't want to be with me. Shirley's words. I couldn't understand why he didn't call. At night I would stand in the park opposite his house and look at his bedroom window, thinking as hard as I could, "Call me, call me, call me." I knew he could hear me; we were connected. Our minds had become connected when our eyes had locked together while he'd watched me stroke myself on his floor.

The months stretched by and I wrote poem after poem about missing him. I drove around and around his house, playing The Blue Car Game. Night after night. Day after day.

And then I saw something that fractured my heart.

One night, as I was on one of my many drive-bys, I looked in the upstairs window of David's house and saw a woman. In his bedroom. He was dating other women? Why not me? I started to cry. I ditched the car around the corner and walked back to the park opposite his house. I hid behind a bush and watched her through my tears, mesmerized. But what did I expect? He was a single man. Cute, a doctor. A good catch. My poor heart. I watched as one arm went up and then the other. What was she doing? Oh, she was putting on pajamas. Pajamas? That somehow cheered me up. Who wears pajamas when they go to bed with a guy?

As the days went by, the pain in my heart became almost unbearable. I *prayed* to David, *please see me, please.* The image of him constantly floated just under my thoughts. I could feel his arms cushioning me as I moved through air. An endless refrain of his name chorused through my brain. David this and David that. The ache for him had overpowered me.

The pain was so pure it was like the silencing of the song of songs, which was silent to begin with. I knew there had never been any noise between us. There had always been a perfect eternity of nothingness. I hoped I had been more than nothing to him. What could possibly be beyond the pain of ending nothingness? Would the grief kill me?

I drove around his house more and more. I played my game. He loved me.

Another day I stopped my car in front of his house. Yes, he existed: this was his house. It existed. He lived there. I had proof. I saw it. And he had a life. There was his recycling bin! I pulled a hat low over my identifiable red hair, got out of the car, and walked past the bin. I hungered for details about him and how he lived in his life.

The bottles, cans, and paper in the bin beckoned to me; they revealed clues about who he was. I squinted at it closely as I sauntered past. Oh look, he drank Merlot. And Tropicana for breakfast. He made tuna sandwiches. And read *McLean's Magazine*. The need to know more overpowered me. I turned on my heel and sauntered back. And then I picked up the whole bin and emptied it into the trunk of my car! Bits of paper that he had touched floated down like feathers.

"Hey, what are you doing?"

I jerked around, startled, and saw a neighbour who'd stuck his head out of his window. I panicked. Oh my god, how embarrassing. I'd been caught doing a really strange thing. This much I knew.

"I'm looking for something." That sounded so feeble. I tried again.

"He took something from me and I want it back."

I didn't know why I said that, but I did. It sounded pretty good. I then turned on my heel as if I had full right to the booty in my car, got in and gunned away.

Shit, what if the neighbour told David? He'd think I was nuts. I squirmed. Oh well, at least I had bits of him in my car. I drove my treasures home and examined them carefully in my garage. The pain in my heart let up as I imagined myself with David, holding the shopping list he had written as we went up and down the aisles in the grocery store.

Finally he called. I was ecstatic. When he suggested coffee again I agreed readily. As David licked the froth of his spoon I couldn't get my courage together to say, "Lucky spoon."

We talked about all the things people normally do while they drink coffee. I kept looking in the street for blue cars.

At the end of our coffee date David said, "So, it was great seeing you again Kathy. How about lunch next time?"

A blue car went by. See, it worked. Lunch was better than coffee, right? He loved me.

A button hung by a thread on my therapist's jacket and her little dog trembled beside her. I jokingly called it "Fang." I settled into Shirley's couch and caught my breath.

"I wrote another poem last night."

"Let me guess, was it about David? Write poems about other things."

Oh sure. Didn't Shirley know the only thing in the world was David?

"He's kinda on my mind." I loved euphemisms. "I called it 'Distance.'"

I pulled the poem out of my purse and read it to her. I listened to my flat voice grate out the story of me tossing a thousand pieces of him over the back of a ship and watching the sharks attack. I wished I could stop thinking about him. I told Shirley I was obsessing less about David.

"The day you don't mention his name is the day I'll know you've stopped obsessing about him."

"But I feel calmer."

And I did. Driving around his house, now forty times a day, going through his recycling at least once a week, talking out loud in imaginary conversations and playing The Blue Car Game all calmed me down.

"I have some strategies."

"Was your relationship with him sexual?"

I stared at her. I crossed my arms. I had to tell the truth; it was a failing of mine.

"Yes."

The word escaped my lips before I had a chance to think. Shirley mustn't report him.

"You know if you tell me his name I have to report him."

"I won't tell you his name. Please don't report him. I'm in love with him. We fell in love in his office."

"Did you ever have sex?"

"Ah, well, yes, no, not really, well, sort of. It was pretty intimate. He fingered me and I had orgasms. Also, we had mind sex. I mean, I masturbated in front of him while he watched and our minds connected while I talked dirty to him. Mindfucks. Sorry for swearing. But please don't report him. He loves me."

"Okay, I won't report him, but don't tell me his name. That would put me in an awkward position." She yanked at her pant leg—it was riding up her calf.

My body was slowly falling apart. The pain surrounding my thoughts of David was twisting me into a contortion of who I had been. I could barely stand up straight without feeling a stab in my lower back. My right shoulder seized up. I got shingles. I got a cold. I got an earache. I got the runs. My foot hurt. My hand hurt. I limped from appointment to appointment with physiotherapists, chiropractors, massage therapists, and doctors.

I now hated being touched but my body hurt so much I had to get treatment. Needles terrified me, but I went to get acupuncture. I lay still with pins stuck in me to alleviate the anxiety, the knee that wouldn't work, the body that was now crooked.

I had to get David out of my mind.

I travelled to Nova Scotia, looking for blue cars all the way. One Saturday night, when I was sure David was on a date, I began cutting down trees and dragging them into a fire. My energy drove my arms and legs like I was possessed. I was desperate to get David out of my head.

I could hear coyotes howling in the distance through the shreds of mist left behind from a hurricane that had swept through the day before. I could hear the foghorn moaning as the sea rose and fell like the breathing of a far off spirit. I cut balsam after balsam and heaved the small trees into the fire. I indulged myself in the lovely memory of nuzzling my cheek against David's chest and nesting with him in the song of songs The pain of knowing I would never hear this nothingness again hissed into the night air as the smoke from the fire rose into the sky.

I was driven to clear the land. I knew I would have to cut down every tree in Canada before I could get rid of the ache of knowing I would never hear the song of songs again. This was my beginning, this night, as I chain-sawed my way through the forest.

He had said on our last date that he would never be my lover. In fact, he had almost shouted it. At the time I thought he protested too much, that it was his fear shrieking, but on that Saturday night, the truth began to smoke around my soul. I cut down tree after tree and threw them on the fire in the middle of nowhere. I watched the smoke curl up and around the moon as sparks stung my skin. I barked back at the coyotes, throwing my voice upward so the sound would travel over the hills. I moaned with the foghorn as pain grabbed at my heart.

I knew I had gone mad and giggled.

How did I get it so wrong? I was sure I had heard the song of songs in his arms. How could I have made such a horrible mistake? I could not bear the reality. I grunted and moaned and howled as I dragged trees across the yard into the fire. The mosquitoes stuck to the sweat on my skin and I could see smears of black ash and streaks of blood in the flickering light. I was doing everything I could not to die from the pain. So, I cut down trees on a Saturday night in the middle of nowhere while he fucked yet another chick in Toronto.

I shouted into the forest, "I clear bush. He fucks it."

I laughed hysterically at my joke.

I drove back to Toronto and hunkered down, waiting for David to call. Things were adding up and infiltrating the chaos in my mind. So many things with him had gone wrong. During our last date on a patio I felt *he,* not me, was under a frozen lake and I only had an hour to chip through the ice to find him. I tried to be funny and make him laugh. At the end of the date he stood up and hugged me. I kissed his skin above his tank top and felt his chest hair against my lips. He hugged me some more and I kissed him again. It was as if the world had melted around us and we were swimming once again in each other. And then suddenly he was pedalling away on his bike, a nonchalant wave goodbye. No promise of anything at all.

I lay on my bed beside Richard, wanting to touch him and not knowing if I could. I was torn in two directions and wondered what it sounded like to hear a heart break. Pain was sitting so heavily on my chest that I could feel the weighty pressure collapsing my lungs and pushing at the center of my universe. And finally I heard it. A breaking heart sounds like the wind in reverse. Like a wave not finding land. I could hear the milky way spinning backwards. It sounded like the song of songs erased. It sounded like nothing at all.

Richard reached a tentative hand for me under the covers.

"Not tonight sweetie, my asthma is kicking up. I seem to be having trouble breathing."

I went back to Nova Scotia and walked on the beach. I had to get David out of my head. I was desperate.

Even in the expanse of a huge beach and a wide open sky I couldn't get away from him. Reminders were everywhere. The wind caressed the leaves. The sun set the earth on fire. The waves curled softly on the beach. It was him touching the landscape inside me. With every step I took on the magnificent beach I knew I had to erase him from my landscape. I knew I had to look at the land the way I used to, where my god was in nature and nature was a part of me.

As I walked on the wet sand I was determined not to think of him. I would *not*. But it was terrifying, if not impossible, because I knew that removing him from the landscape in my mind would rip my soul out of me. I started to cry, the wind drying the tears on my cheeks.

I rummaged frantically in my backpack for my Swiss Army knife, opened it and gripped it in my fist as I fell to my knees. Wailing, I struck at underwater rocks, trying to sever him from the ocean, from the land, from me. I heard the metal slice through the water and clank against the stone.

I was cuckoo.

It was cold in my therapist's office. Dark gray clouds hung in the sky and wind rattled the sliding glass doors. I could hear the electric heater whirring in the waiting room. The little dog was curled up beside Shirley, not trembling for once under a thick duvet. Go figure. On really cold days Fang was warm. The Bully was looking at me intently, her head cocked on one side.

I could tell something was coming.

"You've been telling me for over a year that you are less obsessed with David. And yet you are still doing that blue car thing and looking at his house from the park and driving around his house. So I don't think you're over him at all. Am I right?"

I couldn't meet her piercing blue eyes. Shirley was on to me. She knew I wasn't a woman in transition. That I was bonkers. Way too hard for a regular doctor to deal with. I had failed. I had let her down. Shame welled up inside of me. I was stupid and worthless and now Shirley was going to tell me she couldn't help me. I didn't deserve to be helped. I knew it. I was a very bad person. I knew that for sure.

"Yes."

"I could give you a little white pill and you would feel better. You would also gain weight and lose your sex drive and not feel much else."

"I don't take pills. My mother died taking pills. They frighten me." I was mumbling.

"Well, you know I don't like prescribing them and I know you don't like taking them. That's why I suggested drinking St. John's Wort. I think that worked. You don't seem depressed to me. Other things, but not depressed."

"Yeah, it worked. So does eating salmon and turkey. They increase seratonin and tryptophan levels in the blood to ward off the debilitating effects of depression." I said the last sentence as if I were reading it out of a medical journal. Shirley laughed.

"For over a year you have only written one poem that had nothing to do with David. This one."

She tapped the wall behind her head where she had hung my poem about land and sky meeting in the prairies and how the air sounds when they connect. I had written it for Shirley because a truly mystical moment had blanketed her office when she had described how she felt about the prairies to me. I had tried to capture the power of her feelings for them in the poem. And perhaps I had. There it was, after all, on her wall.

"I know. He's on my mind a lot."

"More than a lot."

So she knew. "Yeah, all the time. I can't get him out of my head."

"There's a new treatment for post traumatic stress disorder caused by traumatic experiences. It's called EMDR. EMDR stands for Eye Movement Desensitizing and Reprocessing. Obsessive compulsive behaviour is a symptom of post traumatic stress disorder, and I think this treatment might help you. I think you were traumatized by a doctor being sexual with you while you loved your husband. Would you like to try it?"

"Tell me more about it."

"There are a few psychiatrists in Toronto who are doing the treatment. It's supposed to remove the fear from frightening traumatic memories. You still retain the memory, but it doesn't seem so bad when you think about it. It helps your brain waves calm down. Something to do with filing the memories away into healthy memory. The therapist waves fingers or lights back and forth in front of your eyes."

Just what I needed. Voodoo medicine.

I was now forty-five years old and if the rest of my life was going to be worth living, I had to get help. My poor children needed their mommy and although I was doing my best, I wasn't really there for them any more. I remembered how I'd already driven around David's house three times that day and it was only 9:30 in the morning. How I'd gone through his recycling bin just yesterday. How I'd tried to send David mental messages to call me from the park two nights ago. I remembered the night I'd howled at the moon while burning bush.

I knew I was bananas.

"I'll try anything."

CHAPTER 13

I WAS TOTALLY FLUMMOXED. Staring at the sheets of paper didn't help. I picked them up and read them over, yet again. I ran my fingers through my hair and rubbed my eyes. This was the sixth time I had read them. I was trying to make sense of the directions for a test that my new therapist had given to me.

Shirley had given me a list of psychiatrists who had EMDR training, but all of them had huge waiting lists, some of them five years long. I was potty right *now*. So I called a private therapist on Shirley's list, Maggie Pope, who could see me right away. It was going to be expensive, but I figured I'd save on gas if she could get me to stop driving around David's house.

After my first meeting I knew I liked Maggie. And I wanted Maggie to like me. Maybe, if I did well on this test, she would.

But I just couldn't grasp what I was meant to do. I used to make up tests, and now I couldn't even do one? I hated being stupid. I had to figure it out. I was meant to do something with a slash on a line. Why couldn't I get it? What did the slash mean? I saw the line; it was below the question. I took a deep breath and read the directions again. The words kept jumping off the page. The paper became a shade of gray and then suddenly turned a startling white. Then the words changed shape. Maybe the light was too bright. I turned out the dining room lamps. I squinted at the pages and the words stopped dancing around. I put my face right up to the paper and read them, one by one, with my finger underlining each one. I whispered them out loud and tried to string them together in my mind so they'd make sense.

Finally I had all the words memorized. I closed my eyes and repeated the instructions to myself. "Mark on the line below each question how often you feel the answer to the question."

I held the paper up and looked at the line. On the right there was a one hundred percent, on the left, a zero.

Ah ha! I got it.

I said, "If I mark the line on the right, that means 100 percent of the time. If I mark it on the left, then hardly ever. Okay, now I know what to do."

The very first question was a no brainer. Good thing, considering it appeared I had no brain.

I read out loud, "Some people have the experience of driving a car and suddenly realizing that they don't remember what has happened during all or part of the trip. Mark the line to show what percentage of the time this happens to you."

"Ha!" I laughed. "That's easy. One hundred percent of the time." I marked the line. Then I whispered, "She'll thinks I'm nuts." I quickly erased my slash.

I paused. "I *am* nuts."

Then I shook my finger at an imaginary listener, "But I don't want the therapist to know I'm nuts."

I very carefully put my new slash on the line at 90 percent of the time. The only thing I knew while driving my car was how many blue cars I'd seen and whether or not David loved me. I knew I babbled away to myself in imaginary conversations with him. I hadn't told Maggie about these little glitches in my mind and didn't want her to know. I wanted her to like me, not be frightened of me. I wasn't going to tell her about The Blue Car Game. Or The Chat Room. Not yet anyway.

Then there were a few questions in a row that established, as far as I could tell, if someone was one step away from being a bag lady. I read them out loud.

"Do you look down and seem startled by what you are wearing because you didn't remember putting on those particular clothes? Do you find your shopping cart full of things that you don't remember putting there?"

"I'm okay with that one," I muttered. I put down just two percent of the time. There was nothing specific about finding my watch in the flour canister when I was in university. How long had this *really* been going on? Since Tippy disappeared?

Then I gasped. The next one was a doozey. "Some people have the experience of feeling as though they are standing next to themselves or watching themselves…"

"How did they know I do that?" I asked no one in particular.

I used to joke with my darling David how I never felt alone. How I totally understood the idiom, "I am beside myself." How I would watch a movie, a horror flick, and be the central character. Did that make me crazy and unlikeable? I decided it did, so I put my mark close to zero.

"I better be a bit more honest than that." After another stab at minimizing the truth, I marked my slash at about fifty percent of the time, softly singing Joni Mitchell's refrain, "two heads are better than one."

Then I babbled, "Some people have the experience of looking in a mirror and not recognizing themselves."

Jerking back and gasping when I walked by my hall mirror would no doubt qualify for one hundred percent on that one. It was so true. "I never know what I look like. I am always startled by the woman in the mirror; it's never me. If it were me, then I'd have to recognize myself, wouldn't I?" So I hedged the truth and put my slash on the line at ninety percent.

I spoke the next question. "Some people have the ability to ignore pain."

I was really good at that. I'd walked around with a dislocated shoulder from a skiing accident for a full day before I got help. That day I kept looking at my arm in astonishment, as if not being able to move it was a betrayal. I'd hardly felt the pain. I put down fifty percent. Too many nineties would tip the therapist off that I was slightly, if not wholly loony.

Then I read aloud the next question. "How often do you experience yourself talking to yourself while you are alone?"

At that I burst out laughing.

My level of upset was like a volume knob, going up and down with my state of distress. Talking to myself calmed me down. It was my secret world. I could control it. It was where I could be perfect for David, where we were in love with each other. I put down one hundred percent of the time. Then I held it up and looked at it.

"I'm not a gospel shouter!" I whispered animatedly while I was erasing. "Sure I shout, but just in The Chat Room. And never to god," I pointed upwards, "just to David. That makes it okay, right? Right. I jiggled my slash a little over to the left, to about eighty percent of the time.

"There, Maggie won't think I'm whacko." I said quite loudly. Then

I put my finger on my lips and said, "Sh-h-h."

Maggie was looking at my test and talking. I was trying to stay focused and hear what she was saying. I kept looking around the room. The pictures frightened me as they zoomed in and out from the walls.

"This test measures how much you dissociate. That means how much you feel you are not in the present, that you are not here." She was putting marks on my test. I hoped I wasn't totally nuts.

Maggie went on while she ticked through my answers. "Dissociation is a symptom of post traumatic stress disorder." Maggie added up the figures and did some math. I looked up at her, "You've measured very high, with a good portion of your time spent being dissociated. That means you often feel like you're not here. I'll give you the test again in about a month to see if you're responding to the EMDR therapy."

So Maggie knew that I was not here. The bad news was that I was crazy, but the good news was that perhaps this treatment would help me out of my deep dark hole. I looked carefully at Maggie, who was now sitting back. Hmm, I thought, she doesn't seem to mind that I'm literally out of my mind.

And then Maggie wanted to know more of my history. I felt like a puppet as my mouth flapped open and shut with the story of my childhood, my life, and my being in love with David.

"Okay," Maggie finally said, "Now we'll do some EMDR therapy. I want you to think of a time where you felt safe."

I settled down; this seemed simple enough, so far we were just talking. Easy. Except I didn't understand the instructions. "How do you mean, 'safe'?"

"A time when you felt relatively calm and at peace."

I racked through my brain. Safe? I had never felt safe. I trolled through every memory neuron to come up with a scenario. I didn't want to disappoint Maggie. Surely there was some point in my life where I felt safe. Surely there was.

There wasn't.

Panic gripped me. What was I going to do? I couldn't even do the very first job of this therapy. I had to have this therapy. It had to work. But I wasn't going to lie. I sat looking at the therapist and she looked back at me, waiting, her hands patiently clasped in her lap.

Shame and embarrassment washed over me. My shoulders hunched up and I felt my insides begin to tremble. I had made it through my whole terrible story about my childhood without crying, and now I felt a flood in me open and spill into the room. I started to cry, the tears rolling uncontrollably down my cheeks. Would I drown?

"I'm sorry." I covered my head with my hands. I had to hide my face. "I can't think of a time when I felt safe. I have never felt safe. I can't do this. I'm so sorry."

I hung my head as shame clutched my heart.

As I was looking down I imagined Maggie standing by the door, saying, "You're too stupid. Everything that's ever happened to you was all your fault. You know that. I can't help you. You are beyond help. You don't deserve to be helped anyway. Away you go."

I raised my eyes slowly to see if Maggie had shut my file and was waiting by the door to usher me out. But no, she had moved her chair right in front of mine. Maggie sat very still, her hands in her lap and her feet close together. She was leaning forward slightly, her eyes looking at me intently.

Was she going to touch me? I kept an eye on her hands. But she was sitting absolutely still. Maggie seemed to be totally unfazed. I decided in that moment that nothing startled her. Maggie was utterly solid. I had to trust someone and decided right then it would be her. Her hands were staying in her lap. She didn't get up. She didn't shout at me. She didn't move a muscle.

"That's okay, Kathy. Let's do it this way." Maggie was speaking gently and softly, as if she were addressing a wounded animal. "Why don't you imagine what it would feel like to be safe? What it would feel like to be calm. Get a picture in your mind of a place where you might feel peaceful and calm."

Maggie's eyes were an anchor for me as I floated around in my mind, trying to imagine what it felt like to be safe. Finally I imagined myself standing at the top of a cliff overlooking the town of Huntsville, Ontario. Lion's Lookout. I imagined the sun shining on me and birds singing in the distance. I saw the pine trees rooted to the side of the cliff. I felt myself calm down as I looked over the town into the wide open air.

"Okay, I have a safe place."

"Keep seeing the picture in your mind. Follow my fingers with your eyes."

Maggie moved her fingers back and forth in front of my eyes. I followed them the best I could and felt my eyeballs rolling back and forth in their sockets. I kept the image of the view over the town in my mind the whole time. Although I felt that staring at someone's fingers moving in front of my face was a bizarre thing to do, I could feel my blood moving warmly through the veins in my arms. It felt so soft. Fluid. I could physically feel my body relaxing.

Maggie stopped moving her fingers. "What's happening now?"

"There's a fabulous view overlooking the town of Huntsville from a cliff. Lion's Lookout. It's beautiful and calm." I rubbed my arms slowly and whispered, "My blood is moving in my arms."

Maggie smiled, leaned forward, and continued with a number of sets of EMDR. Each time I elaborated on more and more of the details of what I noticed in my safe place: the trees, sun, birds, water. I began to feel calmer and noticed I was breathing more deeply.

"How are you feeling now?"

I felt almost giddy. I had a safe place! "Pretty good, relaxed."

"You notice that your safe place is on the edge of a cliff?" Maggie smiled as I shrugged ruefully. "That tells me how bad it's been Kathy. Don't worry, you'll feel better soon. Practice going to your safe place several times a day before our next session. I want to be sure you are good at going there before we start working on your traumatic memories."

While I drove around David's block that night, I practiced being in my safe place.

CHAPTER 14

ALICE, A FRIEND OF my daughter Margaret's from school, was also best friends with David's daughter, Miriam. We all lived in the same neighbourhood so it was not surprising that I would eventually meet up with someone who was friends with David's family. The three girls would sometimes hang out together, but now Alice was sitting across from me in a restaurant, stuffing her mouth with pasta. Her parents had asked me to take her out for lunch once a week because she was acting up and I seemed to relate well to her. I didn't mind because I found Alice to be an engaging young woman, smart but unfocussed, which was pretty typical for a kid of fourteen. Alice chattered away about her best friends, including David's daughter, Miriam. My ears perked up when Alice let the bomb drop that David now had a steady girlfriend, a woman much younger than he was, and everyone in the neighbourhood thought she looked silly with him.

"What's she like?" I was trying to keep my voice light. So the woman in PJs wasn't a one-night stand.

"Uh, your typical bleached blonde bimbo. She works for the government."

"You don't like her?"

"Cindy's pretty nice to Miriam, but you know, like too nice, like she wants to be her friend."

"Oh yeah, I know what you mean. What's her last name?"

Alice chewed her pasta, "Heffner."

So, David was seeing a girl named Cindy Heffner. Probably wasn't serious. When I got home I looked up her address in the phone book. Good, way across town, no chance of bumping into her.

"Tell me more about your childhood, Kathy." Maggie looked at me carefully. It was our third session.

"There was this time when I was little, about thirteen, when I stood in front of my mother's bedroom door. I had had an asthma attack and was standing in the hallway, waiting to see if my medicine had worked or if I needed a shot of adrenaline. Anyway, I was really cold in my nightgown, shivering, and it was dark and I could hear this…"

I hit one fist against my palm.

I looked at Maggie to see if she registered what it meant. Maggie nodded.

"My mother was being hit by Lynn. I told you about her. Lynny-poo." I wrung my hands and leaned forward. "I could hear my mother being hit on the other side of the door."

Maggie asked me, "What is your negative belief about yourself from that incident."

"I just stood there. I went back to bed. It's my fault." The terrible word caught in my throat. "I should have saved her."

"And what would you like to believe? What would be the opposite of it being your fault?"

I looked at Maggie as if she were from another planet. Maggie had said "opposite." What? That it wasn't my fault? That's the answer? It was a ridiculous notion, but I knew it was the right answer and wanted to please Maggie.

I said questioningly, "That I was a child and I couldn't do anything about it? That it wasn't my fault? That I'm safe now?"

Maggie said, "How much do you believe that? Your beliefs are measured on a scale of one to seven, with seven being completely true and one being completely false."

Ah, so Maggie knew it was ridiculous. I wailed, "I don't believe it at all."

"So a one." Maggie jotted on her paper. "How were you feeling as you stood outside the bedroom door listening to your mother get hit by Lynn?"

"Helpless and terrified."

"Your feelings are measured on a scale of one to ten. If ten is the highest level of disturbance and zero is no disturbance, where would you put how helpless and terrified you feel now as you think back on this."

I remembered the event and felt helplessness dissolve the muscle control in my arms. "Ten."

Maggie wrote that down too.

"Where in your body do you feel helpless and terrified?"

I rubbed my arms up and down and whispered, "Here. My arms. And here," I touched my neck, "My throat."

"Okay, now see the picture in your head of you standing outside your mother's bedroom door, listening to her getting hit. Be aware of thinking it was your fault, that you felt helpless and terrified. Focus on the feeling in your arms and throat."

I looked at Maggie as she said this. Did she know what she was saying? Fear sliced through my veins from my heart to my fingertips. Could I recreate the memory in my mind's eye? Would I live? But I remembered my resolve to trust Maggie and watched her fingers as they began to move in front of my face.

I saw myself waking up with an asthma attack and creeping into the bathroom for a slug of my yellow licorice-tasting medicine. In my mind, I could hear the clink of the glass bottle on the porcelain sink. I remembered freezing in my nightgown, covered in goosebumps as I stood in front of my mother's door, waiting to see if the medicine worked or if I would have to get a shot of adrenaline. I heard the sound of flesh hitting flesh reverberating in my ears. I saw myself slinking away from my mother's bedroom door and tiptoeing into my bedroom. I recalled how I had lain down on my bed, listening to fear hissing in my ears and putting me to sleep. Maggie stopped moving her fingers and told me to take a breath in and let it out.

"What happened then?"

I told her the whole story, everything I had seen in my mind, omitting nothing. Maggie listened quietly and didn't move a muscle. I ended with the hiss of fear in my ears.

"Where do you feel it in your body?"

"What? The fear?" How did Maggie know I had razor blades coursing through my veins and my skin was burning off my arms?

"Yes, the fear. Where do you feel it in your body?"

"Uh-h," I made up my mind, I would tell Maggie. "I, uh, have, I have razor blades cutting inside my veins and my skin feels like it's burning off."

Maggie nodded as if this were an everyday occurrence. "Focus on where you feel it in your body."

She moved her fingers back and forth in front of my eyes while I focused on the veins in my arms. On my burning skin. My mind wandered back to the little girl standing in front of the bedroom door. I saw her listening. She was so cold, so little, so thin, so frightened. I gathered her in my arms and held her. I could feel her little body trembling as I wrapped my arms around her. The little girl cried and cried as I told her it was okay. It wasn't her fault. She was just a little girl. Maggie stopped moving her fingers and told me to take a deep breath in and let it out. I did.

"What happened then?"

I told her about rescuing the little girl from the landing. Tears fell out of my eyes as I spoke, I felt so sorry for her that my heart hurt. I told Maggie what I felt in my heart.

"Focus on the pain in your heart."

Maggie moved her fingers back and forth in front of my eyes again as I felt the pain in my heart. I replayed in my mind how I had rescued the little girl from the sound of my mother getting hit. I gathered her in my arms and took her to the view from the top of the hill in the town of Huntsville. When I got there, the young girl danced out of my arms and floated happily away into the sunshine. Maggie stopped moving her fingers in front of my eyes and told me to breathe in and let it out.

"What happened then?"

I told her what I had seen in my mind's eye and Maggie again asked me how my body felt. I touched my arms in amazement and started to laugh. Holy smokes! How did that work? The razor blades were gone. I had no pain in my heart. The skin on my arms had stopped flaring up.

The memory of standing outside my mother's door flowed past my mind's eye and nothing happened in my body. I made a smacking noise with my fist in my hand, a sound that I had never been able to tolerate. "Just testing," I said to Maggie. But nothing was happening inside my body. I wasn't frightened.

I was astonished. "How did you do that? How long will that last? Will it come back?"

Maggie leaned back in her chair, her hands quiet in her lap. "We don't really know how it works, but the introduction of bilateral stimulation such as eye movement allows people to process traumatic memories in such a way that they no longer cause the same distress."

It sounded like a foreign language to me, but I sure felt lighter in my head. I was ecstatic and made my next appointment right then on the spot. When I got out of Maggie's office I stood in the doorway, waiting for my eyes to adjust to the glare off the snow. I watched the traffic whiz by in the street and listened to wet tires sloshing through the February slush. The sound flowed around me like waves on a beach. For about ten seconds I did not have David in my head. I was actually *here*.

Suddenly it hit me like a ton of bricks that I wasn't playing The Blue Car Game. After just three sessions with my new therapist I had stopped looking for blue cars, something I had done twenty-four hours a day for almost two years. I'd get better!

I had to tell someone the fabulous news. Who could I call? Certainly not Richard, he didn't know about The Blue Car Game. Marion. My neighbour. I knew Marion would understand the importance of this moment.

"Marion!" I shouted into her answering machine, "You'll never guess what. Never in a million years. I came out of Maggie's office after my first EMDR treatment and guess what?" I hollered joyfully into my little cell phone, "I'm not playing The Blue Car Game!"

I paused and looked at my phone, "Oh, sorry, that was a bit loud." I lowered my voice, "I am not playing The Blue Car Game, Marion. Just in time for my coffee date with you-know-who tomorrow. Love ya. Bye!"

CHAPTER 15

THE PHONE RANG. I put down the iron. I was getting ready for my date with David, pressing out the wrinkles of a shirt while trying to press out my sadness for being demoted from lunch to coffee. "Hello?"

"Hi, Kathy," his unmistakable accent flowed through the wires. "I have to cancel tomorrow's coffee. A conference."

What? I held the phone away from my ear and stared at it. The night before and he cancels?

"Oh, David, that's okay." Not.

"I'd like to reschedule for lunch two Saturdays from now. If you're available."

"Let me check." Hmm, he was leaping over Valentine's Day. I rolled my eyes upwards and counted to five. "Yeah, it looks okay."

"That's great. Same time, same place?"

On our previous date we'd had lunch at a cute café on Bloor Street. He'd looked like hell while he reassured me he was getting his life together.

"Sure, works for me."

Promoted back to lunch! I hung up almost hysterical with giddiness. No more idiot coffee! He *was* in love with me. I danced around the room, my freshly ironed blouse clasped to my chest, getting wrinkled again. The dog looked at me, his head cocked to one side.

I drove around the city blowing up red balloons and tossing them one by one into the back seat of my car. I laughed when I caught the eye of other drivers as if sharing an inside joke. They looked away quickly. At home I tied the balloons together. I was going to attach them to his car! Happy Valentine's Day! So funny!

At five a.m. I crept out of bed so as not to wake Richard and drove over to David's house. I did a quick drive-by to assess the situation.

"So, his car is here. The lights are out. Her car is gone. Wait a minute. It was here earlier. Hmmm ... did they have a fight? On Valentine's Day? Maybe they broke up."

I parked two houses down from his and looked up and down the street before getting out of the car. No boogey men. I grabbed the balloons by their strings and shushed them when they bounced together as I shuffled towards his car. I was as quick as I could be in the cold, tying the balloons to his wipers with fumbling fingers, looking up every two seconds for that nosy neighbour. Finally I was done and scurried back to my car, giggling away.

I wanted to admire the effect from a fresh perspective so I drove around the block and then slowly back up his gray street. The balloons were bouncing wildly, tickling the belly of the grim February morning. I drove past them hooting.

They were hilarious! He'd love them!

When my family woke up I made them a Valentine's Day breakfast, placing foil wrapped chocolate hearts at everyone's places. Then I quickly drove Jamie to hockey and after tying up his skates, took off for David's house. I parked across the street and finally saw his face looking out his bedroom window. I instinctively ducked, then peered over the dash to see him marching towards his car. Something metal glinted in the sunlight. A knife? Scissors? He started jabbing at the balloons, one by one. I watched his elbow swing back and forth, stabbing systematically. He was so angry. I could tell.

I sat in my car and sighed. I started to whisper, "What's wrong with you? You're an idiot." And then I spoke louder. "Next week when I see you? Boy oh boy, I'll say, "You must be the only man alive who wouldn't be tickled pink by a pretty woman putting red balloons on your car. I just wanted to make you laugh." I wanted to get my lines down pat. So I shouted the same line again, "You must be the only man alive who wouldn't be tickled pink by a pretty woman putting red balloons on your car. I just wanted to make you laugh. That's what I'll say. I'll practice in The Chat Room."

I rested my head on the steering wheel. Then I dashed back to the arena, just in time to see Jamie score.

I was waiting for David in the little café, sitting in the sunlight as it blazed through the window. I picked up the menu and tried to read the entrees. The words vibrated on the page and my throat tightened. Jesus, I wished that would go away. So inconvenient. Suddenly there he was. I glanced at my watch. Ten minutes late.

My chair scraped against the floor as I stood up. It toppled under the weight of my winter coat. I grabbed at it and set it straight. I lost my balance and knocked my hip against the table. The water spilled. David held his arms open for me to hug him. I stepped on his foot.

But then his cheek brushed against mine and he kissed it.

I couldn't breathe.

"Sorry I'm late, I decided to have a shower after karate this morning." His wet saliva felt cold on my cheek and I wondered if it was glistening in the sunlight.

"Well, I guess I should be grateful then." I gestured, "Sit. Sit. How are the kids?"

We gabbed about nothing in particular. The room swayed around me as I tried to keep calm.

He ordered for the two of us and then, of course, brought up the red balloons. "Did you put balloons on my car for Valentine's Day?"

So predictable. "Yes." I knew what was coming.

"I didn't like that."

Of course not. Damn. I thought I was so ready! But no, the mere thought of challenging him caused me to dissociate and I watched myself from behind the lens of a movie projector. I wasn't here at all. But I had rehearsed my lines and damn it, I would say them.

"You must be the only man alive who wouldn't be tickled pink by someone doing something as silly as putting red balloons on your car by a pretty woman."

There! I'd said it! Sort of. I thought I had blown it a little. Did it make sense? I turned my head so he wouldn't see my lips move as I said it again to myself. It wasn't quite right. A man a few tables away thought I was puckering my lips at him and winked back. I jolted my head back towards David. I waited for him to say something. He was looking down at his plate. Oh what a darling. I stroked his hand.

"I have trust issues," he said.

"Of course you do, your marriage broke down. That's okay. Next year I'll just give you a rose. An interesting rose, but just a rose."

We said good-bye in the cold spring rain. He leaned over and kissed me, again on the cheek. "I'm looking forward to seeing you again."

I looked up at him and said, "Does this mean we're boyfriend/girl-friend?"

"Absolutely NOT!" he shouted.

I took a step back. Holy smokes! Time stood still as I watched a small drop of rain splatter his glasses. I wanted to reach up and wipe it off. Silence hung in the air like it does after a car accident.

"Well, if that's the case, I don't think we should see each other again."

"Fine." He strode off toward his blue car.

My world lurched noisily around me. Why had I said that? I knew I couldn't live without him. I staggered to my car. The next thing I knew I was putting my keys into my front door. I ran upstairs to my office and grabbed the phone.

"David, it's Kathy. Listen, if I could press an undo button I would. It's just we had such an intimate relationship and I miss it."

"You're the one who said it." He was accusing me.

"I know, and now I'm taking it back." I was begging him.

"I only want to be friends. We're just friends. Nothing more."

"Okay David, just friends."

"I'll call you in a little while."

We hung up and I replayed his "Absolutely NOT." He had protested too much. He loved me, no doubt about it. We had progressed from morning coffee to lunch; perhaps dinner would come next. I began the long vigil for his next call.

I drove around his house thousands of times, babbling away. Waiting was driving me crackers. I went up north and walked on the frozen lake, hoping I would fall through the ice. I imagined myself making naked snow angels, the harsh granules scraping my skin, my body heat melting the ice, until I plunged through.

I wanted to die. I waited months and months for him to call.

Finally his soft voice cascaded through the telephone line and flowed through me like a warm river. He asked me out for dinner. We had moved from lunch to *dinner*! "Dinner, dinner, dinner!" I sang into my kitchen. My dog barked happily and nosed his dish across the floor.

David and I were seated on the noisy terracotta tiles of a romantic Italian restaurant on College Street. He always picked places with bad acoustics. The noise clattered off the walls and I tried to ignore it as I scattered my three leaves of high-priced baby greens around my plate, trying to make them look like more. I was starving from my run before dinner but controlled my urge to inhale the tiny wisps of lettuce.

"Can't believe they're charging so much these days for salad." I tossed a bruised leaf from left to right and finally speared it.

"I know. Prices seem to have gone up." David reached across and stabbed one of my bits of lettuce. I almost forked him. "Good dressing though," he said while chewing.

Looking at me across the table he said, "So, what have you been doing lately?"

"Oh the usual, taking care of kids, running errands, going out with friends." Driving around your house. Going through your garbage. The usual.

I tried to read what was lurking behind his glasses when he asked, "Sure you don't want a glass of wine?"

Fuck. Couldn't he remember a single thing about me? I hated wine. It tasted like anti-freeze.

The entrées came and went, and we exchanged stories about kids and families. The dinner was over way too fast and during our hug good-bye on the street I tilted my head up for his kiss. I barely felt it. It was a small sort of chicken peck, just slightly off the corner of my mouth. Had he wanted to kiss me and missed? How do you miss?

My ears were ringing from the noise of the restaurant as I drove away. Although the date was over, I was still talking to him out loud, saying all the smart things I should have said to him so he would love me. "Did you read about the Kyoto Accord last week?" and "I hear that the quality of Toronto's drinking water is equal to, if not better, than bottled." "I understand asthma rates are skyrocketing in children."

Every now and then I banged on the wheel and sang, "I'm nuts, I'm nuts, I'm fucking nuts." I thought it was funny and laughed at myself. Then I thought it wasn't funny and despaired. Oh my god, what was wrong with me?

Later that night I cracked open a beer and sat in my office, dreamily savouring the memory of his arms wrapped around me after our dinner. Then I whispered, "Why the hell didn't we kiss?" And then, "Why didn't you kiss me?"

I jabbed at the air with my finger. "Why not?" And then louder, "How do you miss? How do you fucking miss?"

The kids were at school and Richard was off at work. Hooray! I was alone! And it was garbage day! I zoomed down to David's, hoping against hope that I'd get there before the garbage truck came. I screeched in front of his house, pitched his recycling into the trunk, and squealed back home, delighted with my catch. Then I dumped the pilfered contents onto my kitchen floor and poked through it, heart pounding. I touched every single piece of paper as if it were an extension of him. I prayed no one would come home. What on earth would my kids think? They were older now and would know I was doing something weird. Richard, who put the garbage out, never noticed the extra amount he had to drag from the garage to the curb, thank heavens.

I rifled through his discarded mail, his hair dye box (!) and his bank receipts. But then I found something really interesting. "Hmmm, what do we have here?"

Hidden in the corner of an old magazine envelope were a thousand tiny bits of torn up paper. A jigsaw puzzle. What was he hiding? The pieces fluttered to the kitchen floor and I moved them around and around until they slowly fell into place.

Bit by bit, I could read whole sentences. I was reassembling an information sheet from a drug store! I started to breathe very hard when the word Viagra appeared. A hundred excuses for David flew to my lips.

He had prescribed Viagra for himself! Were doctors allowed to do that?

I leaned back on my haunches and let out a long sigh toward the ceiling, my eyes closed. Questions whirred in my brain.

"I don't get it," I whispered into the air. "He didn't have any trouble getting it up with me. That's for sure."

While the refrigerator hummed I remembered how his penis had felt like a steel rod pressing into my back as he had held me like a baby. I shivered.

While I gathered up all the little pieces of paper and threw them in my garbage, I puzzled over what might be going on in his head and finally gave up. I couldn't figure it out. Was it my fault? I washed my hands.

I didn't believe in Viagra. He shouldn't be putting a chemical in his body that would no doubt harm him one day. I grabbed my car keys. I had to go to the dry cleaners to pick up Richard's shirts. "I'll tell him on our next date not to take it." I got in my car and laughed as I pictured the scene. "Oh, hi David, just happened to be going through your garbage and I came across all these tiny bits of paper. After I spent hours and hours assembling them, I discovered you prescribed yourself Viagra."

On my way to the cleaners I just happened to swing by David's.

Finally, after a few months, he called. Again he asked me out for dinner.

We were sitting in a sexy French bistro on Queen Street West. I hugged my feet against the electric heater that ran below the windows under the table. He had been on time and had kissed me in that cheek-licking way that he had. I would have to talk to him about that. One day. When we were together.

But that meant I'd have to leave Richard. I'd never do that.

I played with my napkin and screwed it up into a tight little knot as I tried to screw up my courage to talk to him about the Viagra business.

"Sometimes I think some medicines are pretty dangerous and prescribed pretty flippantly. Take the birth control pill. It's responsible for strokes and cancers in women and yet it is the most prescribed drug to females. And now we have Viagra for men who have a sexual dysfunction. If you're not turned on, you're not turned on."

David took the bait. His voice rolled across the table like the soft waves on my beach. Oh god, I loved him.

"But people have to get on with their lives. Just last week I prescribed it for a middle-aged male patient who'd been through a nasty divorce and wanted to have an intimate relationship with a woman, but couldn't."

Oh my god, he was talking about himself. Ah, so things weren't going well with his pajama-wearing girlfriend. I tried not to gloat. He didn't have those problems with me, no sireee.

"Even so David, if the guy isn't getting it up, then maybe he needs to wait some time to allow himself to heal from his marriage breakdown. It's so typical. Guys get a divorce and the next thing you know, they're dating some bleached blond bimbo, ten years younger than they are. It's a set-up for disaster."

"Well, maybe so, but the guy gets a sexy, young wife."

Gets? A guy "gets?" I couldn't believe what I was hearing. He was talking about men using women. Oh my god. What a jerky thing to say.

CHAPTER 16

MARION WAS LEANING BACK in her chair at her dining room table, watching me carefully. "So, what are you going to do about Blackwood and Valentine's Day this year, Sky?"

"Ha, you've remembered last year. What a debacle! No balloons for him this year. No way." I rolled my eyes. "No, I promised him a flower. I got it this morning."

"What'd you get?"

"I hunted everywhere for something unique. I couldn't just send him tulips or roses. That's not what forty-seven year old women do. We're maturely elegant. I found him a single white tropical Christmas Rose. It's fabulous."

"I've seen them, they're huge. You getting it delivered? Won't it freeze?"

"No, they delicately laid this beautiful pearly white flower into a large tissue lined box. And then they wrapped more white tissue gently around it for protection."

"You're still nuts about him, aren't you?"

"Oh yeah. I signed the card T.M.D.—Truly. Madly. Deeply."

"It sounds gorgeous, but isn't it a bit obsessive?"

"Of course it's obsessive. I'm in love! It *was* gorgeous, Marion. He'll love it. They tied a thick white ribbon around the box, made a pretty bow and placed it in their refrigeration unit. It was beautiful. I can just imagine him unwrapping it. Lifting it out. Cradling it in his hands." I looked dreamily into space.

"I get the picture," Marion frowned. I shrugged.

Before making a special Valentine's feast for Richard, his favourite, pesto pasta, I drove down to David's neighbourhood. As the setting sun washed the cold February day with a clear yellow light, I sat in my car across the park from his house, waiting for him to come home and rescue the pretty flower from the winter frost. Excitement coursed through me as I watched him slowly lift the box and take it inside. He would love it.

The next morning I got in my car and drove over to his house. What had he done with it? I drove around the block and stopped at a phone booth. I dialed his number, just to make sure no one was home. No answer. I climbed the painted steps to his front porch and craned my neck so I could see inside his living-room window.

There it was! I laughed softly. The beautiful Christmas Rose had been placed in what was certainly the wrong vase. It tilted awkwardly to one side and looked precariously close to falling out. But he liked it! Because there it was, its delicate petals glowing a translucent pearl white on his pine dining room table.

Richard had given me candle holders in the shape of hearts. I loved them.

Two weeks later I opened my mailbox and pulled out a letter addressed to me. As I peered at the writing my heart sank: it was David's small script. What now? I sliced the envelope open with my finger, knowing I was going to be chastised for something I had done. I was getting tired of always being bad. My eyes darted over his words and anger bubbled in the pit of my stomach.

"He's lying to me." Fury raged in me as I read the letter. "He's lying to me. He didn't like the flower? He threw it out? What? It was still on his dining room table this morning. I saw it. It was still there. Two weeks later!" I poked my finger at the letter.

And then came the zinger. I read it out loud, "...before we all go on a holiday, of course." I said the sentence again, imitating his smarmy, patronizing tone. "Before *we* all go on a holiday, of course."

Rage hammered my skull as I squished the letter into a tight little ball. I punched the air with it, and whispered loudly, "THIS is how you tell me you have a girlfriend? You bastard! Where are your manners? You can't tell me to my face?"

Then I pitched the letter into the garbage and started to cry. After a few seconds I pulled it out of the garbage, flattened it, and tucked it into my pocket.

I burned dinner and helped the kids tidy up the kitchen. I was a phenomenal actress, laughing and asking them animatedly about their school day. As they disappeared one by one to their rooms to do homework, I gathered up my coat and shouted merrily up the stairs, "Off to get milk. Back in ten."

I pecked Richard on the cheek as I dashed by. He looked up from the paper.

I yanked my car door open and rammed through the dark to David's house. I got out and fell instantly on a glassy patch of ice that had flash frozen when the sun had gone down. I looked at my hand in the lamplight and saw blood dripping down my arm.

I didn't care and beat his door with my fist, spraying it with my DNA.

He opened it, chewing the remains of a mouthful of his dinner. His lips curled into a sneer. "What are you doing here?"

His sweat pants were too short.

I waved the letter under his nose and seethed, "Is this how you tell someone you have a girlfriend? By letter?"

He snickered at me, his patronizing superiority twisting his lips into a dismissive jeer, determined to place the blame on me, "Well, you gave me a flower."

"For heaven's sake David, it was for Valentine's Day. This," I hit the letter with my hand several times, "is pathetic. This is something you do in person. Where are your balls?"

"You seem angry."

Duh.

"Can I come in?"

"No."

Helplessness fed my rage. Blood dripped down my sleeve. I let the letter fall to my side and turned down my volume a notch. Cold wind whistled into his house through the open door. I knew Mr. Environmental would be pissed off at the loss of heat. I stared at him and he stared back, arrogance flirting with the corners of his mouth. In the end I won. He finally held the door open wide enough for me to squeeze through.

And then he did the weirdest thing I had ever seen someone do. I watched in horrified fascination as he staggered back and flapped his arms up and down. Like a demented drunk bird, his arms beat at the air as he lurched backwards. And then he scraped at his chest, as if trying to pull off something terrifying.

Was he stoned? I remembered him saying "I smoke dope." I sniffed the air. Nothing. Was he drunk then? I wasn't sure. I tried to glance into the dining room to see if there was a glass of wine at his table. I couldn't see one—the flower was blocking the view. But I could see that he had been eating out of a green plastic bowl. Pasta of some kind. The noodles were glued against the sides.

When he had stopped flapping his arms and finally perched against a door frame, I said, "Look, all you have to do is be honest, David. Don't lie to me. I know you liked the flower. Don't say you didn't."

I flung my arm in the direction of the dining room. "It's still on the table for Christ's sake."

I was gathering steam.

"And why do you go out with her? Everyone knows she doesn't turn you on."

Oh no! Would he know I'd gone through his garbage? David's eyes bulged out of his head, as if his anger were pressing like a fist inside his cornea. I had touched a bit of a nerve, oh my.

"I'm not going to comment on the health of that relationship."

Like it had nothing to do with him?

"And just how old is she, David?"

His mouth clamped shut on his answer. I watched our dinner conversation from our last date register in the furrow of his brow. He suddenly flung open his front door and puffed out his chest, pointing to the street.

I desperately needed to rescue this very bad situation.

"Look, let's not fight. David. Let's both apologize and make up. I'm sorry I barged down here all upset, I should have waited to cool down."

I waited for him to apologize. Then I waited some more. I gestured with my fingers to prod him on. Finally he opened his mouth.

"I'm sorry too."

"For..."

"For sending that letter."

"And..."

"For lying about the flower."

There, he said it.

"So, are we friends now?"

"Okay. Just friends. Nothing more. Those are my terms."

Same old, same old. I said nothing.

He held open his arms and I pressed my face against the squeaky polyester of his too- tight sweatshirt. I kissed him on his neck and waited for the beating of his heart to slow down. This was just like the good old days. When I stood back we were both calm. "So David, what happens next?"

"I'll call you and we'll go out for a nice dinner."

I'd better pin him down. "When do you have in mind?"

"Early May?"

"Did you like that French place? I did."

"Yeah, we'll go there."

"It's a date."

I tripped over the cracked flowerpot outside his front door and stumbled down the peeling wooden stairs, drunk with euphoria. "That went well."

As I drove home, the image of him flapping his arms up and down as he fell backwards replayed in my mind. What on earth was that about? Was he terrified of me? Was it me he was trying to scrape off his skin? Whatever had happened in his marriage sure had scarred him. He was petrified of how deeply he loved me. That must be it. I'd talk to Maggie about it at next week's appointment.

I was at the end of my rope waiting for David to recover from his disastrous divorce and be ready for true love. I needed things to move along. A letter. I'd write a letter to Cindy. Good plan. I'd pretend I was a well-wishing friend who didn't want her to waste another minute of her life with someone like David. When she lost her looks, out she'd go, just like his first wife. I knew Cindy was being used by him. "You get a young, sexy wife." That's what he'd crowed.

I drafted a letter, printed it, and drove across town to Cindy's flat. As usual, I jabbered out loud while I drove. I put my phone on the dash so if anyone saw me, they'd think I was on speaker-phone. I was going to save Cindy from a life of misery with David. Me? I was used to his kind of treatment and could handle it.

My wheels bounced into the sidewalk outside Cindy's house and I turned off the ignition. Now or never. I trotted up the walk and flicked the envelope through the brass slot in her door. The letter floated lazily down onto a pile of junk mail.

My heart beat crazily in my chest as I stumbled back to my car. I had done it! I vowed I would never tell anyone. Ever. No one. Even if my nails were being pulled out. But maybe the letter would save Cindy from an unfulfilled life with David. And maybe David would then be with me.

Finally it was early May and time for our date. I sat at the same booth we'd been in last time. The waiter hovered over me, his silver tray held like a frisbee. David was late. I looked at my watch and played with my napkin. Should I order a beer while I waited? No, too uncouth. I smoothed out the tablecloth.

I picked up a spoon and looked at my reflection. I watched my face distort like a cartoon figure going through a wringer. I drew flowers in the condensation on my water glass with my finger. I licked my finger and then worried about Hepatitis C.

The waiter came back. "Do you want anything? Perhaps a drink while you're waiting?"

"No, thank you. My date must be tied up. But I'll wait just a bit longer." I was getting self-conscious. Where the hell was he?

I finally left the restaurant and stood forlornly in the street. I called his house. No answer. I waited ten more minutes. I called his house again. I called my answering machine. No messages. I called his house again. I looked at my cell phone in disbelief. I whispered as I walked towards my car, "He's just forgotten. That's all. He's gone to karate. Oh you silly boy, did you forget?"

I got in my car and drove to his gym. My hands shook as I clutched the wheel. There was his car! What a little nut he was for forgetting.

My legs felt like a marionette's without any strings, moving in directions I couldn't control as I stood in the doorway of the gym. My eyes searched the moving sea of white uniforms and grunting men until I finally found him in the first row. His bald spot was my first clue. The second was his name embroidered across his back.

I tapped the shoulder of a guy in the back row. "Sorry to interrupt. Could you get that guy, David, for me?"

"Sure."

I watched as the student walked towards David and spoke to him. David's head zipped around and his eyes blazed angrily at me.

I plastered a demented smile across my face as he paced towards me.

"Did you forget our dinner? It was tonight…" my voice trailed off when I saw his glowering face. I edged backwards into the foyer.

He followed me, spitting out words. "I sent you a letter. Didn't you get my letter? I sent it last week."

Now what was he doing? I watched him in disbelief. David kept bowing his head at me, as if he were still in the gym and I were his sparring partner.

"What letter?" I said. His head bobbed up and down. "I'll resend it."

I hated his letters.

I whispered, "What did it say?"

He was bowing crazily and shifting from foot to foot before he delivered his fatal punch. His voice had become corrosive acid.

"You sent Cindy a letter."

Oh, God, he knew about the letter to Cindy. My skin began to disappear. I was dissociating. I had to lie. Nobody could know about that letter. I couldn't lie. But I had to.

"I don't know her address. I don't know her last name. I don't even know what she looks like. How did I get it to her? When did I get it to her? I've been out of town most of the month." At least that was true.

"I don't know what to believe."

"Well, next time ask me."

"You're embarrassing me at my gym."

David turned on his barefooted heel and stomped through the metal doorway back into his class.

Not to be outdone, I stage whispered to the back of his dirty uniform, "You're embarrassing me in my life. My LIFE! You stood me up. In public."

I wondered if the pitying eyes of the waiter counted as "public."

I slumped in my car and tried to control my breathing. I was having a major panic attack. My arms had disappeared. I rubbed them. "Oh fuck. No arms."

I shook my head in despair. "So, it's fast food. How life can turn on a dime. One minute you're all tasted up for French cuisine and then lo and behold, you're galloping towards a hamburger."

After wolfing down my burger I hustled back to David's house and knocked on his front door. I could see him in his upstairs window, the setting sun reflected in his glasses. I called him on my cell. I watched him through the window, watching me. He didn't answer. I left a message, "I really want to see you. I really want to sort this out. Please. I can't bear to think of you not talking to me. Call me, please." Oh, I was begging. The relationship was slipping away from me.

Two days later, David's letter arrived. My heart beat in my throat as I ripped it open. The letter contained everything he had said at the gym, plus it said he wouldn't get together with me anymore and he wouldn't read my letters. He had handwritten at the bottom, "I am sorry you did not receive this in time. I sent it on April 22nd. I am relieved you are not behind this harassment, however I have decided that the trust in the relationship is broken and I cannot see you any more."

I ran my fingers over the ink and pressed the letter against my heart. Dry sobs shook my shoulders. When I reread the letter again, I looked at the date at the top. It said April 28th. Right, he wrote it on the 28th and mailed it on the 22nd ?

The guy was such a liar.

CHAPTER 17

SOMETHING HAD GONE VERY wrong with my skin. I sat on the edge of my bed, rubbing my hands up and down my thighs. Definitely couldn't feel them. I took a pin and touched the point to my leg. And then to my arm. I watched the skin pucker around the sharp point of the pin. "I can feel that." I put the pin down and touched my arm lightly with a finger. "But not this."

My breath came in hollow gasps. "Why did you touch me? All over my body? Did you want to own me?" My voice rose. "You carved your name into my flesh. You branded me. Like I was an animal. I've seen people with scars. They sunburn really easily. You think I'm going to let the world see hot flaming 'Davids' all over my body? No way. I'm going to cover my skin up."

And then I wept. "How did it happen David? Your touch was like the soft foam on the edge of a wave. When did it turn into razor blades?" I rubbed my arms as pain lay heavily around my heart. I held my head in my hands and sobbed. "Why David, why? Why did you carve up my skin? Because it felt good? To you? Did you like it?"

I took a deep breath and lifted my head high. "Boy oh boy, if I knew then what I know now, I would have run and run and run away from you. Anything to save my skin. Ha, that's a good one, 'save my skin.'"

For weeks and weeks my skin hurt and was numb at the same time. I wrote about razor blades every night, tears streaming down my face. All I wanted was to get my skin back to normal. But by summer it was completely gone. It felt like it had burned right off my bones. I decided to go to Nova Scotia to try and heal.

As I was walking on my lovely beach, I imagined that my dry white bones were in a pile, smouldering. One night I wrote five poems called "Bones" while drinking beer.

I knew I was upset; I was talking to myself a mile a minute.

"Oh God, I wish I'd known. His hands were so hot. I didn't know they were burning the flesh off my bones. He left me with nothing, nothing but a goddamn pile on the beach. And now the bones are burning up. I see myself walking around them, crying, my aching wails smoking a dark column of pain high above the sound of the sea. Oh God, I am so ashamed of myself for not noticing the smell of burning skin until after he had gone." I couldn't bear the pain. I gulped my beer and got another. I tripped on the rug.

"It's not true. Is it David? Surely you love me." I thought about that for a long time and then got yet another beer. "Of course you do. Silly girl. You'll see him again. He'll say yes. Because he loves me. All you have to do is ask. Just call him." I calmed myself down. I had a plan.

When I got back to Toronto I left him a lighthearted message. It was just a lover's spat, right? We would kiss and make up.

"Hi David, it's Kathy. Sorry about that misunderstanding. I'd like to get together with you so we can sort this mess out. Give me a shout. Love ya, bye."

Then I waited for three days. He didn't call me back.

I was sitting in front of Maggie. It was confession time. "I keep driving around his house. I can't help it. I have to do it. The kids are safe, I mean, they're old enough to be left alone now. And I don't think they know I'm doing it. Richard comments about my gas bill sometimes, but I don't think any one knows, except, of course, you, now."

"Why do you have to do it, Kathy?"

"I don't know," I wept. "And I have conversations with him. Out loud. While in my car. I call it The Chat Room."

"Sounds like you're keeping yourself really busy. Sometimes people do that so they won't think about something else."

"Yeah, like the pain of him not wanting to see me."

"Do you cry when you drive around his house?"

"Yes. All the time. "

"So what's the pain about that you are trying to get away from? And what's the pain about that you are creating?"

"What? I don't understand your question."

"When you're driving around his house and talking to him and crying, does that pain remind you of any other pain?"

"Oh... Yes, it feels like the same pain when I was in his office after he turned me on and then did things to punish me because I was."

"Sometimes people create painful situations because they're comforting. They feel safe."

"So I have created a fantasy relationship because it causes me pain? And the pain gives me comfort? How sick is that?"

"Well," Maggie smiled, "It's what you have to do. Because you're the one creating the fantasy, you have control of it. And that control gives you back some of the power you lost while in his office."

"How did you know I felt helpless?"

"Victims are helpless."

Victim? I felt the blood in my veins slow down, almost to a crawl. What did Maggie mean?

"Do you think I was his victim? Victim of what?"

"You tell me."

"That sex stuff? Do you think he was using me? Taking advantage of me?" I sat up very straight.

"I think he abused you."

My world stopped turning.

"Did you always know that? Why didn't you tell me?" I was whispering now. The room was leaning off to the right.

"If I had, I would've lost you. You wouldn't believe me. You wouldn't come back."

"Well I don't believe you now. He loved me, Maggie. Really he did. He told me he did." I paused for breath. "So you think I drive around his house so I don't have to face the reality that I was abused? That is, if I was."

Maggie smiled, "You have to admit, it keeps you pretty busy. How many times a day do you do it?"

I looked down at my hands. "About eighty. I can't count. It's a lot. All day."

"Well, think about what I've said."

I drove straight home. It was impossible to swallow the word "abuse." The next day I drove around his block just three times.

From eighty to three. It was a start.

Every three or four weeks I left David a little message on his machine, asking him to call me. Why didn't he call me back? Was it true? Was it over? But we had been lovers. Hadn't we? No it was abuse. I couldn't face that. But I had to. I refused to believe it. I was too frightened to speak to him directly. Then he might tell me it was over. I wept every night for what he had done to my skin.

I went to Maggie once a week.

"He stood outside the office door. He was being my father. And when he came in he leaned over me and touched me all over. I could see him in the light from under the door. He pretended to take off my pink underwear. I saw his hand pretend to throw it on the ground beside me. And then he put his mouth between my legs and I could see his tongue licking the air and he looked like a lion. His face was in shadows from the light coming in under the door and his teeth had a gap in them like a wild animal's. I thought I was going to die. I thought he was going to eat me. The wall behind him went all shadowy like it was covered in flames."

"What did you feel Kathy?"

"I loved him with all my heart."

"Then why are you crying?"

"Because I was terrified. I felt terror."

"Sometimes when people have been abused, but before they realize they have been, they label their emotions incorrectly. All they know is that they're experiencing a very strong emotion. You couldn't handle the idea that what you felt was fear. Love is easier to deal with than terror. You didn't feel love, but terror."

My head felt tight. "Yes."

"And where do you feel it in your body."

"My arms. And my throat. I feel like screaming. And then he circled away from me and told me to lie on top of him between his legs. I thought I was going to die."

Maggie pulled her chair closer to me. "What is the negative belief?"

"That I'm going to die."

"On a scale of one to seven, what's the degree you believe this?"

"Twenty. It's a twenty." I knew I was going to die.

Maggie smiled gently, "And what's the positive belief?"

Could there be one?

"That I'll live?"

"On a scale of one to ten, how much do you feel this could happen? A one means not at all and ten means you feel it could."

"One."

Maggie pulled her chair close to me, "Get the image of him eating you in your mind. Focus on where you feel the terror in your body." She moved her fingers back and forth in front of my eyes as I relived the event in my mind. My skin burned as my tears flowed down my cheeks. Remembering it was hell.

Over the weeks I told Maggie about the fire burning up my skin. How I didn't exist. How I'd kill myself except that I was already dead. About the hiss in my ears. How everything went crackly inside my head. How I disappeared. How I lived in a world wiped out by TV snow. How I felt underwater. And if I closed my eyes I could see a thousand minnows darting away from the pebbles he had thrown into my underwater life.

The therapy was a nightmare, week after week. I had no idea how much pain it would cause me, but I knew it was worth it. It was nothing compared to the pain David had caused. I had to do the work; I was desperate to escape the spell that had been cast on my life. While getting EMDR from my therapist I relived all the events in his office: the rapes, the dramas, the masturbating, the rewirings, the hugs. It was exhausting.

But I was driving around his house just once a day.

And I was having more fun with Richard.

One day I turned on the bathtub tap and put my hand under the running water until I had adjusted it to the right temperature. I stepped into the shower and let the warm water stream all over me. After I had washed and rinsed my hair, I bent over, soap in hand, and lathered up my legs.

I said to myself, "I am washing my legs."

I looked at my legs in amazement.

Again I said, "I am washing my legs."

Excitement flew through me. I said it louder.

"I'm washing my legs." My voice stuck to the steamy walls and dripped down in rivulets.

"I can feel my legs. Holy shit!" I watched the lather on my skin run down my legs like frothy rivers of whipped cream. I could feel the delicious soft foam caress my skin.

There was a knock on the door.

"Hey Mom, are you okay?"

Oh my God, did Emma hear me swear?

"Just fine sweetie, just fine."

I leaned against the side of the shower stall, crying for joy. I vowed never to forget this moment. I couldn't wait to tell Maggie.

Maggie had saved my skin.

The family's finances were desperate. I hadn't worked for years, but I still needed therapy. There was that pesky TV snow problem. But I could no longer afford to pay Maggie. I decided to call a psychiatrist named Barbara Wiley; if she agreed to take me, her fees would be covered by Medicare. I left a message.

"Oh, hello Barbara, this is Kathryn Curtis. I think it might be a good idea to see a psychiatrist to sort myself out. I really hope you have some space. Thanks."

She called back immediately and I told her I was having a weird problem with my head. To my relief I got an appointment.

"I, um…" I didn't want to sound crazy, but I had to tell Barbara the truth if I was going to get help. "I can't stand being touched. And my head sort of hisses and crackles at me. TV snow. You know TV snow? I get it. In my head. And it makes me want to kill myself, but I don't because I'm already dead. I don't have it right now. It comes and goes."

I watched myself talking to the doctor. "Right now I feel very frightened. There's something wrong with my eyes as well. It's like everything is sepia-coloured. There's a wall of old faded yellow between my retina and reality."

"What are you frightened of?"

"You. I mean, everything."

Barbara nodded.

"I get so frightened I feel like I'm living in a Van Gogh painting. The corners of the walls don't meet right."

I looked at the corners in the room. I felt so desperate.

"I have to get this fixed."

"You can come again, next week, same time."

As I was leaving, the psychiatrist reached out and tucked in a clothing tab that was sticking out of my collar. I shrank against the door frame.

I said, "I really don't like being touched."

The corners of the room moved in and out.

When I got home I washed and washed where the doctor had touched me. I trembled in the corner of the shower, waiting for the fear to leave my pores. That night after making scrambled eggs for the kids and getting them off to bed, I went into my office and started rocking back and forth and whispering to myself.

"I'm sleeping. See? My eyes are shut. I'm in the recovery room. In bed. The heart monitor is quiet. Is that black air? Is there black air coming in under the door? I asked the doctor to put a towel down. To stop it. Shhh. Keep quiet. The heart monitor will go off. Then they'll know you're not sleeping. I told the doctor I can't be touched. I told her. I can't be touched. Shhh. Kathy, you'll set off the monitor. You're okay." I heard myself singing, in some far off corner of my mind, "I'm not here. I'm not here. Man are you nuts, stupid. Of course you're here. You're in the recovery room. And you don't want to set off the heart monitor. There's the doctor. She can't see me." I rubbed my arms and legs. "Can't feel a thing. So I'm probably invisible. It's okay, Sky. You're not stupid. You're invisible. The doctor can't touch you, stupid. Shit. Black air. What are going to do now, Sky? It's coming in under the door. I can see it. Fuck. I'm not here. I'm not here. Shut up, Kathy. God, you're a stupid ... Oh no, she's coming towards me. Didn't she hear me tell her I can't be touched. Hey, doctor lady..." I knew I was raising my voice. "I can't be touched. Back off! There goes the heart monitor. It's beeping all over the place. She's talking. I can barely hear her. There's so much black air. Wish the monitor would shut up. What's she asking me? I can't hear her. She's asking me something. What is it? Fucking monitor. Shut up, will ya? She's asking me what's my name. She's saying, 'It's okay, honey, tell me your name. What's your name?' I just don't know. I don't know. Of course you know, stupid. It's Kathy. No, it's Sky. Tell the doctor your name. That's all she wants to know. She doesn't want to know who you are. That you're a stupid cunt. Stop being so cuckoo." And then I heard myself say my name, quite clearly, "My name is Sky. Sky."

I polished off eight beers. I couldn't stand being crazy. But deep down, even though all the professionals in my life called me Kathy, I knew who I was. I was Sky.

After I finished venting in my office I limped into the bathroom to brush my teeth. When I looked in the mirror I didn't recognize my-self. Forty-eight years old and I couldn't see who I was. I *had* to keep getting EMDR. We'd eat at the low end of the food chain this week. I needed Maggie.

"My face is broken in the mirror."

Maggie nodded. "Hmmm."

Thank god for Maggie. Nothing surprised her.

"I am fragments. Every breath of who I am slices away at my brain like fragments of razor blades."

I knew I was talking gibberish. But I had to get it right. Somehow.

Maggie waited.

"I feel like I am swallowing glass." That was simpler.

"You sound frightened of the truth."

I began to sob, "I love him. I can't bear to be without him. I need him. He loves me. The pain is slicing me into fragments. He abused me. No he didn't. I can't recognize myself in the mirror. If I do then it's me."

I watched as Maggie moved her mouth. I forced myself to listen, to make sense of the words.

"What's the negative belief?"

"I can't live without David but I can't live with what he did to me." I paused and said ruefully, "This is a rock and hard place."

We laughed and Maggie began yet another EMDR therapy session.

After my appointment I got into my car and looked in my rearview mirror as I pulled away from the curb. My clear brown eyes looked back at me.

"There you are! You're back. Maggie just saved your life."

CHAPTER 18

ITOOK MARGARET AND Jamie to the Adirondacks again for their March Break. As I drove along the 401 towards Kingston, the word "abuse" swam just under my thoughts like a slow shark, its bubbles breaking on the surface of my mind and disturbing my hopes that David still loved me.

I felt that my deep pain was the same ancient pain that had forced the mountains to come crashing up through the rocks and dirt of the earth's crust. As the tires hummed, the land around me suddenly went haywire. I could hear the bones of rock break as the pressure from below forced the mountains skyward. While driving through the fractured earth, I marvelled at the beauty of the hills and valleys cradling the broken bones.

And then I pushed my foot down hard on the gas to get out of the landscape of a splintering skull. Margaret and Jamie giggled in the back seat. Was I crackers? You betcha.

My mind slowly let go of David's constant presence as my world became safer to live in. It was a roller coaster recovery. Every time I faced a little more of the reality of what had happened to me, I would relapse into a state of extreme anxiety. But by early summer I was beginning to accept that I had been abused. Well, not really. He loved me, but I was a lot better now. I could read. Not books, but a newspaper or a cereal box.

One day I was slowly reading the paper and came across an article about a psychiatrist who had "re-parented" his patient and lost his license to practice medicine. Hey, I thought, that's just what David did to me. He cradled me in his arms like a baby. Oh, how I loved that. Except for the erection part.

I read the article hungrily and made a note of the name of the place that had removed the doctor's license. I'd known about reporting.

But to whom? Here it was. The College of Physicians and Surgeons of Ontario.

I talked it over with Barbara, my psychiatrist. "I think I'm going to call the College and find out if they think I was abused. If I was, then I'll report him."

Barbara never said much, partly because I motor mouthed the whole time, but this time Barbara was very clear: "What you are proposing is a very gruelling process. I don't think you should do this just now. It will take a lot out of you. Don't do this. Not now. I repeat, do not do this now."

Whatever.

The next day I called the College of Physicians and Surgeons of Ontario and was connected to their intake person, Hanna Turner.

"I want to know if I've been abused by a doctor." My heart was in my mouth.

"Did he touch you?" Hanna's voice was so kind.

"Yes," I stammered.

"Where did he touch you?" Hanna sounded so patient, so gentle.

"All over."

"Where specifically."

"Everywhere."

"Can you name the places he touched?"

I wasn't an idiot. I felt like shrieking. Everywhere meant *everywhere*. There was not an inch of skin on my body he hadn't touched. I took a breath.

"I don't think he touched between my toes. Everywhere else."

"Oh, I see. I think you might have a valid sex complaint. There are different levels of sexual complaint decisions. Did he touch your clitoris?"

I whispered, "Yes."

Hanna and I were in a large room with thousands of pot lights jabbing my eyes as she explained the reporting process to me. "This is the room where complaints are heard. It's sort of like a court." Hanna swept her hand around the room.

"Oh." My head swam with all the details about reporting and committees and time-lines and rooms. I didn't take in a single word

Hanna Turner was saying. The room vibrated and sepia bled across the ceiling. What was I doing here? I loved David. He didn't abuse me. Barbara had been right.

I was talking to Marion, now a very good friend. "I can't report him. I love him. It was my fault anyway. We made sure of that, it was in our contracts, that it was all my sexual energy, my hand guided his hand."

Marion sighed. "Okay, think about this. If a man is pointing a gun at a woman and the woman says, 'Go ahead, shoot me,' is the man guilty of murder?"

"Of course he is. You're not allowed to shoot people."

"Same diff, Sky. You're not guilty. You became very sick because of him."

"I almost died." I pointed at the corner of Marion's kitchen. "You know, the corners don't meet. Weird huh?"

"Other women should be protected from him."

Marion's lips were pressed so tightly together they were bone white.

Fear slowly left me and other emotions crept in as I got tons of therapy from my two therapists. I saw Maggie every now and then, either because I couldn't be in the here and now, or because I was *still* doing the homework David had told me to do. The homework where I was to masturbate daily and fantasize about a better ending to the day when he put his erection in my face and I couldn't touch it.

And I saw Barbara once a week and read her poem after poem about being in a recovery room with black air coming in under the door. In some of the poems I had no legs and was in a wheelchair. In others I would try and leave the room but would step into outer space and freefall into a black hole.

But between the two therapists, the hissing air around me finally quieted down to the point where I could sit in a room and listen to what people were saying. The atoms in the air seemed to be joining back together again.

But at night I would have terrible nightmares of David performing oral sex on me, his eyes piercing through the smoky gloom of madness as his tongue flicked between my legs. Fire smoked around his mouth as his two devil teeth glinted like metal traps. I would scream until I woke up. My husband would say, "There, there," and wrap his arms around me. I hated being touched and tried not to scream some more as lions flitted across the backs of my eyelids and I shook between the clammy sheets.

As time went on, I eventually no longer needed the soft cradle of melancholy to hold me. The constant presence of David seeped out of me into the land and the land seeped back into me. My god was returning to the living landscape in my heart. Every now and then pain consumed me because David had salted my earth and destroyed my religion. Months later, David was almost completely out of my mind.

I stopped going through his garbage.

I found the now-yellowed article about the woman who had reported her doctor to the College of Physicians and Surgeons. Her name was Ann Foster. I held up the photograph of the woman and wondered if Ann would talk to me. I called the author of the article at *The Free Press* and explained that I too had been abused by a doctor, in much the same way as Ann Foster. I asked how I could get in touch with the woman. Three days later I was listening to Ann's voice pounding down the telephone line like wet cement pushing down a chute. I knew I had met with a force.

"What's the asshole's name?"

Wow. "Ah," I hesitated, was it safe to say his name? "I haven't told anyone his name."

"Typical," Ann snorted, "You in love with him? Still?"

How did she know? "Ah... well..."

"After what he did to you? C'mon. What's his name?"

What's made *her* so aggressive? I twirled the telephone line in my fingers. "What happens if I tell you?"

"Nothing. Listen, all victims—and that's what you are—all victims of sexual abuse fall in love with their perps. They have to. To survive. Of course you want to protect him. All victims protect their perps. But look, you're here. You've survived. So, what's his name?"

My blood rushed to my hands. All victims? I was doing normal stuff? Feeling I had to protect him? Relief rained all over me.

"David. David Blackwood." There, I'd said it. I'd told someone.

"Let's get the fuckhead." Her laughter sounded like a tornado bashing against the sides of the Grand Canyon as it boomed down the line.

I watched the corners of the room collide.

"He won't know what hit him, the slimy piece of shit. There's a train coming down the track and it's aiming at him."

Ann roared with glee.

I said, "Oh."

Three days later Ann and I met in an upstairs patio on Bloor Street near High Park. The early fall sunlight cast sharp shadows across the plastic tables and I tried to read the menu as the words jumped off the page. I finally ordered from the specials on the blackboard.

Ann was talking. "So, you're going to take on the College?"

"Take on the College? I did meet one person there. Hanna Turner."

"Oh, their poor excuse for a support person?"

"She seemed nice enough to me."

"Listen Sky, the College is not your friend. Repeat after me, the College is not your friend. Get it?"

I said, "Oh."

"There is absolutely no defence for what that schmuck did to you. And the less defence there is, the more the defence will attack you and make you look like you're crazy. The College won't fight back. They'll say it's wasting their time. Be prepared for that."

Again I said, "Oh."

"Let's get down to business. You're going to have to write a Letter of Complaint. That's where it starts with the College. And you'll need a lawyer to start a civil suit. You'll sue the prick as well, right? Call mine. Say I sent you."

She thrust a business card at me. So I was starting two processes: reporting him to the College and suing him in a civil suit.

I took the grimy coffee-stained card and tried to read it. It was the name of the same lawyer Maggie had recommended. Jeff Duffy. Fancy that! Karma. I tucked the card in my wallet.

"What's in a Letter of Complaint?"

"Don't worry, I'll help you. But if anyone asks if I helped you, you say no. They'll think I influenced you, they'll call it a conspiracy, they'll twist it around. Those defendants can be ridiculous."

Ann snorted into her glass.

"What's a defendant?"

"I used to get that mixed up all the time. You are the plaintiff. He is the defendant."

Ann had dragged the word "plaintiff" out into a long whine. "You are com*plain*ing."

"I get it." I knew I would never again get the two words confused.

Ann reached into her plastic shopping bag and pulled out a jumbled pile of paper.

"Here, you'll need this. It's a copy of the Act. The *Regulated Health Professions Act*. RHPA for short. It governs the behaviour of doctors."

Ann slapped it on the table and shoved it towards me. I eyed the coffee stains and grease marks with trepidation.

"Should I get a tetanus shot before I touch this?"

Ann hooted. "Yeah, it looks like I wiped my ass with it."

"I'll copy it and get it right back to you."

"Naw, don't bother, keep it. It's worth shit. Toilet paper, that's what that Act is." Ann gestured the air with a large paw. "Besides, if I need to look up anything in the Act I'll go on the Internet. All you have to do is type in RHPA. Read it and write your letter. As I said, there's a train coming down the track..."

I laughed right out loud with Ann and stashed the Act into my briefcase.

A week later I was ready to know the truth. Did he love me, or was it sexual abuse? This time I'd call David when I knew he was home. I could face whatever he was going to say. No more of those monthly messages of useless twitter. I'd been doing that for at least a year and a half, ever since he stood me up for that dinner on Queen Street. My heart quivered in my chest as I sat at my desk. I started to dial his number and hung up, my hands shaking. "Oh, for fuck sake," I whispered. "Stop it."

I calmed myself down by using an EMDR technique of putting one hand over one eye and then switching to the other hand and eye. One eye, then the other. I did it slowly five times. There, I was ready.

I dialed his number.

His soft voice breezed down the wire.

"Hello?"

"Hi David." I held my breath.

"Who's this?"

What? He didn't recognize my voice? "Kathy," I choked.

Click.

He'd hung up on me.

Click? I held the phone in front of my face and looked at it. The click echoed in my ears. Did I get that right? *Click?*

I stood very, very quietly while I looked out the window. I could feel my blood softly moving through me, like a slow gentle river. I crossed my arms and rubbed them. Good, I could still feel my skin.

I whispered into the dusk, "So, it *was* abuse."

CHAPTER 19

I MUST HAVE PUT the phone down because the next thing I knew I had a pen in my hand and a pad of paper in front of me. I caressed the paper lovingly and wondered why I had never noticed the lines before.

"See?" I murmured. "The blue lines are like the horizon between the ocean and sky." I held the pad in front of my face, tilted it sideways and lined my eye up with one of the lines. It was perfectly straight.

I began to write and talk as if I were explaining something to a young child. "See, I'm writing on the horizon between land and sky. I am so lucky. I can do this over and over again. It's okay, Sky. Everything's okay. Everything on this horizon, this blue line, is truth, beauty, and unity." I sighed in relief. "This is where I live, where I am safe. I can write words on the blue lines. This is what I do. I write. It's okay, Sky."

However, I wasn't actually writing words. Just thousands of loops neatly circling slightly above the line. I was staying alive.

I sang, "Loop-de-loop. Loop-de-loop. Ha ha, I'm loopy."

I was staying alive by dancing on the blue line and looking, in my mind's eye, at the horizon of the sea. Every now and then I gasped for air. Finally I stopped making loops, and wrote, "Why did you hang up on me?"

I knew, of course, it was because he never loved me, because he had always been abusing me. But I didn't believe what I knew. I tried to believe with all my heart that it was because he was too frightened of loving me.

I caressed the page again and wrote about the blue line. Everything was going just fine until my mind swayed slightly off center and I started writing about ashes. Oh god, not ashes again. Swallowing ashes was an impossible job, but swallow them I would. I had to do it in tiny little bits. Some smouldered and glowed and burned on the way down. And some had been doused; these steamed and clumped in my throat. And some of the ashes were as dry as dust. I gasped and I choked and I knew I would get through the goddamn pile of David's ashes if it killed me.

Then I cleaned my whole house from top to bottom.

"What are you doing, honey?" Richard was watching me wipe down the mantelpiece. "It's past midnight."

I hid my tears and mumbled something that Richard couldn't hear.

"Okay then, I'm off to bed. Come up soon, Sky. Love you."

His steps disappeared up the stairs and I whispered, "Love you, too," as I polished the grate with small, circular loops. God forbid that Richard should ever find out about David.

That night I had a terrible dream. It was a dream about me dreaming. I was asleep because I was so sick I thought I might die. I was trying to get well by sleeping underwater in my house. I hadn't locked my doors because I didn't know I should. I didn't understand about thieves and what they could steal. Besides, as far as I could tell, there was nothing to steal because I didn't really exist. I was a dream. So a thief marched right into my house and carved off every inch of my skin from my breasts, the small of my back, behind my knees, between my legs. The water darkened with my blood and I couldn't see. The underwater dream turned into a nightmare.

I begged the thief, "Why are you here? There's nothing left of me. You've taken everything there is."

The thief told me that he loved me, trapped me in his arms and pressed his erection against my bones. I rescued myself by feeling nothing. In that nothingness I discovered peace, love, and happiness. I discovered the truth of who I was. But then the thief pressed his erection against this as well and robbed me of my nothingness. Then he ran away with his treasure and I chased him for years shouting, "Thief, thief."

In this very bad dream I knew I could never go to the police because they would ask me, "What exactly did this thief take from you?"

And I would have to say, "He took nothing, nothing at all."

The police would ask me, "Did you lock the house?"

And I would have to say, "No, the doors were wide open."

And then the police would say, "Asking for it, weren't you."

When I woke up the next morning my head throbbed and I staggered around the kitchen making breakfast for the family. Boiled eggs and toast. I drove the kids to school and then went to Staples where I bought a green portable file box and a box of files. I had a new plan. While I drove home I sang through my tears, "I'm gonna wash that man right outta my hair."

Even though nobody was home, I locked my bedroom door and emptied out my closet of every single piece of hidden paper that had to do with David. I tossed the pieces into different piles on my bed. Letters to him. Letters from him. Therapy Notes. Receipts. Information from his garbage. I neatly labelled manila files with a Sharpie and filed all the bits away.

Then I dumped my sock drawer on my bed and tackled the huge mountain of poems. Thank heavens Richard never put my laundry away. What on earth would he say about this! Hundreds of them filled eight files, one for each year since I'd met him. Every now and then, one would catch my eye and shame would overwhelm me as I read how I wanted to lick him like soft ice cream or feel his hot fingertips steaming on my body. I carried the full portable file box to my office and put it in a corner. I pointed my finger at the box. "I'm watching you, Dr. Blackwood."

That's who he was, *Dr.* Blackwood. The box seemed huge in the corner. "I'm going to write about what you did. A Letter of Complaint." I began scribbling lists and dates of what had happened to me in his office. Every so often I would look at the box and then drag my eyes away to continue writing.

I picked up the kids from school and went on autopilot for six hours. Dinner. Dishes. Dog.

That night I went back into my office with a line up of beer. My mind whirred around the dark memories, trying to make them come into focus. Trying to put everything in chronological sequence. I wrote down all the he saids, I saids. I backed everything up with a column of the titles of what had now become dirty poems. Woven throughout the tapestry of all my memories was a sad thread of incredible disbelief. I was such a fool. Silly, silly me to trust him. I swallowed and gasped for air as I wrote, shards of pain slicing the back of my throat.

I had seen him earlier that day when I drove the kids to school. He was riding his stupid bike. He only rode his bike to work on the days he taught his environmental class at the university. What a hypocrite.

I saw he was riding on a busy sidewalk, going the wrong way on a one-way street. So typical. He didn't see me and rode past. Figures.

I called Hanna Turner at the College. "I am pretty worried about this process of reporting. Does the College have any legal help for victims?"

"Ah," she coughed, embarrassed, and then named a local sexual assault support organization that I could turn to.

So now my green portable file box was at my feet and the piece of paper I was holding was shaking as I read my chronological list of events to the director of the clinic. Self-doubt overwhelmed me while I told my story under her imperious and challenging stare. Did I get it right? Was I lying? I felt like a butterfly pinned to a wall of fault as guilt congealed on my wings.

The director's voice floated above me in a gray confusion of sounds. What was she saying? "Go for sexual impropriety. Misconduct. A lesser charge. He won't lose his license. No way. They'll attack your credibility."

I was disgusted. "What would it take to tip the balance towards sexual abuse?"

She answered, "History. If he's done this before."

"Great." I said. "I'll become history. The first person doesn't count, she's 'history.' The College has a zero tolerance policy, but only if there's *history*?"

Anger flared on top of my guilt and I gathered up my paraphernalia.

I felt jangled as I walked down the gray-carpeted hall and put my hand against the cool wall for support. I carried my silly box to my car through the fall drizzle and was irrationally ecstatic I didn't have a yellow parking ticket glued to my windshield. The meeting had gone on way longer than I thought it would. On the way home I bounced between peals of laughter and screams of "Fuck!"

"It's not right," I shouted in The Chat Room. "Doctors can't use patients. Can they? Can they touch them just like that? Oh my god, are we as barbaric as that? Unbelievable." I laughed and swore. "Surely we protect women when they're ill. I was ill. I couldn't *see* straight." I laughed hysterically. "Is this the fucking Middle Ages? It's archaic." I pounded my steering wheel.

When I got home I found the lawyer's card in my wallet. Damn it, I *would* start a civil suit as well as report *Dr.* Blackwood to the College. My finger stabbed the buttons on my phone. I left a message, feeling like I was begging.

The next morning I turned on my computer. For the first time in eight years I would write something longer than a poem. As I listened to the hum of the machine I felt like the top of my head was blowing off. I wrote one line, "A Letter of Complaint," saved it, and quickly turned the machine off. I gasped for breath on my couch and tried to slow down my breathing.

One eye, the other eye. One hand, the other hand. I put on my relaxation tape and lay down.

One line. Just one line. "Oh my God!" I groaned, "This is going to take months and months to write."

The next day I sat in front of my computer and wrote three whole paragraphs. I described "Flip the Flip," his cute little rape ritual, his "Let me turn you on and then sodomize you," all fun and games.

The days went by and every day I wrote a little bit more in my Letter of Complaint. When I was done, it was 14 pages long. I read it to Ann and as my voice droned on and on, Ann had two double scotches and five cigarettes.

"I thought you said you were a writer. That's shit. It's all over the place and like four times longer than it should be." Ann ground out her smoke.

She snatched the letter out of my hands and started scratching away with the stub of a pencil, drawing arrows and slashes all over. I watched in fascination as Ann massaged my chaos into a readable format. At the bottom she scribbled a list of words.

"Sky, you gotta use headings. Make it look professional, organized. Get them from the *Regulated Health Professions Act*. There are sections where doctors screw up. Things like 'Sexual touch' and 'Behaviour unbecoming of a physician.'"

I went home and found the coffee-stained copy of the Act in my green box. I ended up with twelve headings: He saw me excessively; Physical touch; Sexual touch; Dr. Blackwood told me many details about himself; Dr. Blackwood accepted many gifts from me; He told me he loved me; Dr. Blackwood watched me in my personal life; He engaged in unorthodox modalities of therapy; Inappropriate medication usage; Unprofessional conduct; Verbal abuse; and He engaged me in social meetings away from the office. Then I went through my very long story and cut and pasted like crazy, putting the right information under the right heading.

Three long months after that awful meeting with the legal director, I was almost ready to deliver my Letter of Complaint. I thought about the consequences of what I was doing. If I sent the letter, then for sure I would never get back together with David.

Duh. But now he was *Dr.* Blackwood.

I was having lunch with Marion and said, "But what about Cindy? Dr. Blackwood's's girlfriend?

"Dr. Blackwood? You're not calling him 'David' anymore?"

"I'm trying not to. He isn't my lover. He isn't my friend. I'm going to report him. I just can't think of him the way I used to. So, it's Blackwood from now on. As much as I can remember. It will probably take a while because "David" was such a refrain in my head."

"Well, 'Blackwood' makes sense, it gives you distance."

"But what about Cindy? She will be affected by the Letter of Complaint as well. I don't want her to be hurt. She probably doesn't have the slightest inkling that her boyfriend is an abuser."

"Don't worry about her, Sky. She's a big girl. She can take care of herself. Just do what you have to do. Hand in the letter."

"But I feel I should save her from what's going to happen. She'll be dragged down as well. She shouldn't suffer."

Marion replied, "She might tell him and then you'd be scuppered."

"I know, but I wish I could protect her. And his partner, Dr. Charles. He seems such a nice man. Should I tell him? But then, he must have sensed that Blackwood was doing something odd. Should I warn him?"

"Absolutely not. If Blackwood knows he's going to be reported he'll tamper with the evidence. You know what he's like: he'll *doctor* it." Marion put the emphasis on the word "doctor" so I would get it.

I knew what it meant. I'd been doctored.

I felt so badly about Cindy being hurt by my reporting Blackwood that I resolved to send her a warning email. But I would have to be careful: I didn't want David, no, *Blackwood,* to have any idea he was about to be reported.

I rifled through the file from my garbage collecting days and came up with some incriminating letters from women I thought he'd had an affair with. Finally I had four names plus mine: ammunition. I would let Cindy know about David's multiple affairs!

I pulled up my hood, put a scarf over my mouth and went to a library that had internet access. I quickly set up a Hotmail account with Blackwoodslover@hotmail.com as the address. That would catch Cindy's eye. In my email I counselled Cindy to never trust that schmuck and to ask these five women what he was doing with them while he was married. I included myself in the list. I laughed at my clever decoy. Alice, my daughter's friend, had told me Cindy worked for the government and I'd found her email in their directory. I pressed "send" and crossed my fingers.

I told absolutely no one what I had done. I was so ashamed of myself, but I had to protect Cindy. I knew there was a train coming down the track and it was aiming at Blackwood. I didn't want any other casualties. It was just a few days before Valentine's Day.

No flower for David this year.

CHAPTER 20

FLICKERING ON MY COMPUTER screen was what I hoped was the very last draft of my Letter of Complaint to the College. I'd got it down to five pages. Then I wrote a brief covering letter to my lawyers for the civil suit. It told them my letter to the College was attached, how this letter started the clock ticking on my statute of limitations, would they let me know if they would take on my case, and that I trusted them. I used really long sophisticated words to help me maintain some dignity while I begged for help.

Then I pressed print. I needed to deliver four copies of the Letter of Complaint: two to the College and two to the lawyers for the civil suit. Lawyers collect paper, and I wanted them to have mine. All of it. I stuffed the letters into their envelopes.

Before I put them in my briefcase, I held the lawyers' envelopes to my lips and kissed them. "Please take my case. Please." I had been badly hurt and I wanted justice. I didn't really trust them at all, but I desperately wanted to.

I slid my four envelopes into my briefcase. It was a cloth affair with a zipper and no handle. Cheap looking, but politically correct. I walked gingerly around the briefcase as it lay on my kitchen counter, as if it contained a grenade. Was I doing the right thing? I *could* throw the letters out; I didn't have to deliver them. Then I wandered around the house searching for any telltale trace of my letter: a working draft, a discarded note. It would be a disaster if one of the kids found anything. Or Richard.

Before I went on my delivery rounds an old friend, Fay, came over for lunch. I didn't see Fay as often as I saw Marion, but our relationship stretched back over the years, ever since Richard and I had bought our house. Her kids and mine went to the same school. She knew all about David and the distress he had caused me. Fay was suffering from depression and had just put her dog down. We made a fine, light-hearted pair. She and I crammed tasteless tinned turkey on greasy flax bread into our mouths. We both knew that turkey and flax all contributed to elevating serotonin levels in the brain. So, although our sandwiches tasted like rubberized cotton balls on top of glued wood chips, depression would be held at bay. We ate like troopers.

"Am I doing the right thing, Fay?"

"Sky, a very bad thing has happened to you. Of course you're doing the right thing. If you *can* report him, you should. Not all women can. Look how strong you are. You've even written a letter."

"I guess so."

After Fay left, I pulled on my jacket and ventured out into the howling wind. I headed to the subway with what felt like four ticking bombs in my briefcase. Was reporting him the right thing to do? Why was I so nervous? I was forty-nine years old, surely I should have some self-confidence by now. "I can always turn around," I said to the wind.

I kept listening to myself for negative feelings like melancholy. Or fear. Or revenge. But no, I felt normal. Well, not normal, I never felt normal, but not completely churned up. So, off I strode with purpose and dignity, pressing my way through the howling March gale to the subway. Was the weather symbolic?

I finally found my lawyers' building and glided through enormous rotating doors that whispered and whooshed as they deposited me gracefully inside. I stood and stared around me. The foyer was four stories high and covered with a glittering veneer of polished marble. I was almost blinded by the mirrored light and knew I had to move very, very slowly or I could get hurt. I had to be careful in places like this: they were not designed for people who had the Van Gogh problem. Mirrors were the enemy. Everything was in reverse anyway and then, by a cruel trick of fate, in reverse again.

I felt myself go into a slow motion tai chi mode while the world careened around me. Dozens of people from the business world marched this way and that, all so capable. I admired how they paced along, their polished leather shoes click clicking on the glassy granite. I was not like these bustling grown-ups in their fancy pinstripes.

Not to be daunted, I stared with what I hoped was calm intelligence at a display on the information desk. I was looking for the floor I needed. The display screen was blank. I looked up at the sign above the desk. It said "Information Desk" and I looked back down at the blank display. No information.

So I looked back up at the sign, and the sign still said "Information Desk." I was at the right place. I stood on my tiptoes and peered over the top of the desk. There must be someone behind it. I lost my balance and fell against the display case. It burst into life! Ah ha! A touch screen.

I followed the point and touch prompts, found my floor number, forty-seven, and with this small gem of knowledge, smugly waltzed towards the elevator.

Oh no. There were ten banks of them.

I walked around the large columns slowly, muttering under my breath, "Odd. Even. Odd. Even." Once I had figured out that some went only to odd floors, some to even floors, some to high floors, and some to even higher floors, I could select the one that would get me to forty-seven. All those years of being bored in math paid off. I knew I was odd, but that I'd get even. I snorted at my pun and a guy with a briefcase looked away.

The elevator doors hummed open to reveal an interior of oak-panelled walls. I felt like I was entering a stately home in Olde England. Was I on a National Trust tour? Surely I wasn't really carrying a letter about lying on a dirty floor and doing you-know-what for a doctor. When the doors opened at forty-seven I saw the silky smooth wood of a reception desk curving toward a wall of glass before open sky. The view was incredible: I could see a bank of fog rolling in off Lake Ontario. I thought, oh my, not another bad omen. I had to stop being so connected to the elements.

A woman behind the desk spoke. Of course she had an English accent. "May I help you?"

To the receptionist's inquiring eyebrow I replied, "I have two letters to deliver, one to Dylan Tomlinson and the other to Jeff Duffy."

The English accent said, "The mailroom is on the forty-first floor."

I panicked. Did the elevator stop at forty-one? Did I have to go down to the basement because it was a middle-level-odd-floor? Would I ever find it? I smiled as pleasantly as I could, got the letters out of my environmentally sound briefcase and said, "I'm not very good with elevators."

The receptionist didn't bat an eyelash as she held out her hand for the letters. "Don't worry love, I'll take them."

Maybe I was so informally dressed she thought I was a courier and then realized her mistake. I escaped, cooing and bowing, as I sort of backwards curtsied to the elevators, just to show how grateful I was.

I found the elevator, and plummeted to the ground with ear-popping speed. Then I pressed my body against the wind toward Bay Street where I caught a bus heading north to the College of Physicians and Surgeons on College Street. As the wheels churned under me I chanted, "College on College. College on College." I looked around, but no one had heard me.

When I got there, I asked the security person behind the desk, "Can I please see Hanna Turner, the Intake Coordinator?"

The guard buzzed up while I remembered Ann's words, "The College is not your friend."

"Hello, nice to see you again. Thanks for coming. Please, have a seat."

While I was bending my knees towards the naugahyde, I heard, "Barbara Wiley?"

I froze, knees half bent. Barbara Wiley was the name of my psychiatrist. She had written a Mandatory Report to the College about Dr. Blackwood and his shenanigans. But she hadn't used my name in the letter as his victim; I hadn't wanted her to.

I said, "Yes?"

My heart throbbed in my ears. Probably from the elevator.

"Were you the person in her Mandatory Report?"

"Yes, that was me."

Oh, no! I should have kept my mouth shut.

My first thirty seconds of reporting a doctor had been a disaster. Ann was right, these people were not my friends. I had requested anonymity in Barbara's letter because I didn't want Blackwood's lawyers to know the name of my therapist. If they knew her name, then my psychiatric records would be up for grabs. Not that I had anything to hide. But I wanted some privacy.

I kicked myself. If I had been to Maggie to cure my inability to filter my thoughts before my mouth went into action, I would have sat down, taken a breath, looked at the Intake Coordinator, and said, "I am quite certain that whoever requested anonymity would want that request respected." As we sat in the foyer Hanna's garbled voice floated above my thoughts. I tried to focus on where I was, on being present, and finally regained my sense of self. When she stood up I followed her into a tiny glassed-in prison-type room to talk. I had seen them on TV cop shows but I didn't know they actually existed in real life. They did. What a day I was having. Oak-panelled elevators and prisoner holding rooms.

Despite how things had gone so far, I still had my inner resolve: I knew I was doing the right thing. I watched as Hanna opened my envelope, smoothed out the letter, and read it. Ann had told me that the people at the College were stupid, but Hanna didn't look stupid at all. She looked nice. Her lips didn't move while she read. A good sign.

Hanna looked up and said, "These are very serious allegations."

"I know," I replied.

Hanna tapped the middle of the third page with her forefinger, "The College would focus on this section, 'Sexual Touch.'"

What? To me "Sexual touch" wasn't the most important section. "Unorthodox Modalities of Therapy" was. And so I took a deep breath and said in what I hoped was my most mature voice, "I think the College would be wise to address the issue of unorthodox therapies. This man literally did everything he could to fuck my head. Sorry." My professionalism was slipping. "He was a mindfuck. Sorry. "

"That's okay."

"Dr. Blackwood fucked my head. Sorry. For some bizarre reason, I ended up on the grimy floor of this doctor's office, masturbating in front of him while telling him dirty stories. He rocked back and forth and always said, 'I will be with you in a very powerful way.' I asked him if he was making love to me in his head. He said 'Yes.' It was a mindfuck. Sorry. The mindfuck, sorry, is in 'Unorthodox Modalities of Therapy.' I suffered much more because of what he did to my head." I took a breath and recovered my composure. "I am so sorry for all the swearing."

"That's okay. It's very upsetting."

"You may have noticed that the consequences of his therapy, the impact on me, is not in this letter. This is just about what he did to me. But believe me, bizarre therapy is far more damaging than sexual touch. This guy pretended he was a sexual abuser and acted out rape scenarios with me as the victim. How on earth could that be helpful?"

I rattled on in the glass cage. I was starting to fall apart. "This doctor is a menace. He's nuts."

Hanna responded by calmly saying that reported doctors fall into one of two categories, "They're either mad or they're bad."

"This guy is both," I said as I watched Hanna read on. "I'm worried he will hurt me once he finds out I'm filing a complaint. He's training for his black belt in karate. He pushed me. He shouted at me. He has major anger problems. Do you think I'm in any danger?"

"No, I don't. When doctors get their copy of the letter they usually call their lawyers right away. The lawyers advise them to stay clean, to change grocery stores if they might meet the patient, that sort of thing."

I changed tack. "I think it's very important that he not be given a chance to doctor my file. He is profoundly dishonest. He lied to me all the time."

I remembered my page called "Lies" and his reaction when I read it to him. He was not one of those chaps who took responsibility for his actions, oh no.

"In my letter I have asked the College to exercise its power to seize my file from his office without warning. Do you need me to sign a form or something?"

Hanna said, "It's becoming more common for investigators to go directly to the doctor's office and hand over the Letter of Complaint while requesting the file."

"Yes, but do I need to sign anything to give the College permission, or is what I say in my letter enough of a go ahead?"

"It's probably fine."

"Probably?"

Hanna shrugged. This did not reassure me. "Probably" was not a word I trusted. There was no way on earth I wanted Blackwood to have the opportunity to doctor my file. He was so dishonest. And remembering that, I let it go; he probably already had.

Hanna asked me, "Does he have any idea about this?" She pointed at the letter.

I said, "No, I don't know how he could. I haven't told anyone who knows him." My little foray to the library and that warning email skipped across my mind. Would Cindy guess and warn him? I hoped not.

After I left, I leaned against the building to steady myself and checked out my body for turbulence. How did I feel? I wasn't going to do anything that hurt me. Not now. I had stayed alive, up to now. Cigarette smoke drifted on the breeze and an image of Lynn holding a knife smoked across my soul.

I pushed off the red bricks and headed towards Queen's Park subway station. The low sun bounced off the mirrored Hydro building into my eyes. There was a whiff of spring on the west wind gusting down College Street. The snow had stopped howling about and I knew something very bad was over. Was this yet another message from the universe? For a brief second in time there were no cars in either direction. In the peaceful silence of that moment I knew it had been the right thing to do. But how did I feel?

That night I shut my office door, slumped on my couch and whispered away. So I guess I felt agitated. "Well, well, well, Sky Curtis. What an awful day. Oh dear, that blurting has to go. How can I get more power? I need the ability to take time, assess a situation, say what I want, and keep my balance. When that hearing rolls around I cannot be caught off guard. I can't blurt a thing."

I took a long drink from my bottle of beer. "And secondly, the College is not my friend."

And I drank some more. "So, it's over. Have I done the right thing? Yeah. Yeah, I have. Probably the best thing I've ever done, writing that letter."

I gulped some more beer. "I fought back. Yup. Not a victim, not me. No way. What did Ann say? 'The more action I take, the more power I have.' She's right. I feel like I have *some* power. Good job, Sky."

But I felt awful. I picked up my pen and started to write a poem about flying high enough above what he did to me that I could finally see what it was from this new light. I described how the fiery heat of my pain smoked a thin white scar across the edge of the sky behind me. I wrote about the roaring sound that turbulence makes, about how difficult it is to extract the cause of the sound from the roar because the acoustic fingerprints are so faint. I wrote about how turbulence can alter the speed of light. How I was screaming in pain so loudly because of the light. I called the poem "Turbulence."

And then I sighed with resignation and got up, scrabbled in my purse for the car keys, and headed into the night.

His light was on in his bedroom window. I wailed as I drove by, "I am so sorry. But I had to. I almost died."

I so badly wanted him to hear me.

I drove around the block again and again, with waves of grief eroding the edges of my heart.

CHAPTER 21

I LIFTED THE METAL flap to my mailbox and peered in, wondering if the lawyers for the civil litigation had written me back. Would they take my case? Did they think I would win? I shuffled through the envelopes. There it was! Shiny black lettering on a sparkling gold background leapt off their cream-coloured stationary.

The letter burned a hole in the kitchen counter all day long, hidden in a pile of bills by the toaster. I couldn't possibly open it. No matter what it said, I would be upset. I eyed it as I peeled carrots for dinner. No or yes? Finally I couldn't stand it any longer. I shoved my finger under the flap and ripped it open.

It said yes. YES!

Oh no.

At lunch a few days later, Ann hungrily grabbed the letter out of my hands. I watched in horror as she smudged ketchup in the margins.

While Ann read I shook my head and said, "This isn't going to happen Ann. There are big problems." The lawyers wanted a $10,000 retainer.

Ann put the letter down, just missing a pool of vinegar, and rubbed her hands together. "What are you going to do about the money? Where are you going to get it?"

I just shook my head in dismay. But Ann loved to solve problems. "I'll lend you $5,000 towards the case. I'll need the money back, but you can pay me when you win."

Underneath all Ann's bluster was a truly kind person. "Oh Ann, that is so kind of you. Thank you so much. But they want $10,000. It seems so impossible."

"You'll find the five grand."

"Forget it Ann, not in a million years. But thanks for the offer." I was discouraged.

"What about selling your house in Nova Scotia?"

I immediately saw in my mind's eye where I had staple-gunned a white plastic tablecloth to the wall struts in the bathroom to make "walls."

I smiled ruefully. "I couldn't sell it even if I wanted to."

Ann chewed on a french fry, assessing the situation.

"Oh. I see. You'd better be perfectly candid with Jeff Duffy about the state of your financial affairs. He thinks you're rich."

"Rich? We run at a whole chunk of change in the hole every month. That's what I used to earn from the paper, before Blackwood. We needed that income."

So I swallowed my pride and wrote a letter thanking them for taking my case and outlining the perilous state of my family's finances. I was basically an impecunious client. Ann had told me to use that word and I pretended I knew what it meant. After lunch with her I'd raced home to look it up in the dictionary. I discovered it meant "dead broke."

Perfect description.

I was in my office with an old camp friend, Jane Wood. She was listening to some of my poems, her eyes half shut. Finally, she said, "Sky, you have to start healing. Your poems are full of pain and darkness. They *are* Blackwood."

"But I have been healing, slowly but surely. I was well enough to write a Letter of Complaint to the College. Well enough to start a lawsuit." I felt like I was whining.

Jane persevered. "All your poems are about him. Or to him. Let him go. Get him out of your mind."

I felt my insides twist into a tight little frightened ball. I couldn't let go of him. I would die if I did. "No, you don't get it. It's so hard to explain. Without him in my mind I won't exist. Poems about anything else but him would have no meaning."

"Yes, they would. Look at that tree out the window." I looked. "See it as it is, unto itself. Nothing more. Do you understand?"

I did. Jane wanted me to get Blackwood out of my internal landscape. Well, so did I! Good luck with that.

That night I wrote a poem about the tree and with it I began the final stage of my healing. I drank and whispered and wrote. "Everything I look at is like a painting of a landscape. Blackwood was like a knife that sliced through the painting." I stabbed the air with an imaginary knife. "I leaked through the rip in the painting to the other side of the canvas." I looked up and whispered again. "Into the black..." I stopped to think of the word, "...bloodiness from behind the painting, Blackwood and the pain he caused, seeped all over what I saw, my landscape." I stopped and wrote that bit down. "But if the frayed edges of the painting knit together." I entwined my fingers. "I will no longer be able to seep behind the canvas of the landscape into the blackness behind." I moved my hand as if it were going behind the painting. "And the black pain he caused on the other side will no longer seep from behind the painting to surround my landscape."

I sat at my desk breathing slowly, eyes shut, and went deep inside my mind to where the pain was, to behind the rip in the canvas. I willed the frayed edges to come together and become whole. I forced myself to see just what I was looking at. Just a tree.

"That's it! I get it! I can keep what I see, my landscape, on the canvas of my vision. I can see the tree, as it is, unto itself." I rejoiced. It was a start.

The phone rang and I wiped my wet hands on a tea towel to get it.

"Oh," there was a pause and I could hear rustling papers. "It's Judith Harrison calling from the College of Physicians and Surgeons. Is Kathryn Curtis there?"

Jesus Christ, I thought. What if one of my kids had answered the phone? So unprofessional. But at least she called me Kathryn, not Sky. The College was not my friend, as Ann had reminded me a hundred times, and only my friends called me Sky. I said in my most I-am-not-a-whacko voice, "Speaking."

Judith said, "I've read your letter. It was very well written. In fact, it was the best letter I've ever received. And then I saw that you are a writer, so that makes sense."

"Thank you. I took my time writing it." If only she knew!

"These are very serious allegations and the College is responding to them with seriousness. The College has decided to investigate your allegations against Dr. David Blackwood and we would like to get a statement from you. It takes the better part of a morning, so we'd like to start fairly early."

"No one in my family knows about this, so it'll have to be after they're gone in the morning, around 9:30."

I felt clammy all over.

The investigator said, "How about in two weeks, say April 30th at 9:30. Maybe you'll have some evidence to give us? You need to be aware that everything we have, every record, letter, document, every single piece of paper, his side gets. But everything his side can find, they keep."

I already knew this from Ann. "That's pretty disgusting."

"Yes, it is."

"I've heard he gets an independent law firm to represent him for free and I don't get a lawyer at all. I am just a witness for the College, and the College lawyer is acting for the College's interests, not mine. Well, I should be represented by a lawyer at the College, too. It's pretty disgusting."

"We're trying to make some changes. But yes, it is disgusting."

I offered, "I've got my government health insurance records. Do you know he billed for virtually every single time I saw him, even the very short sessions where all he did was hug me?"

"You have your records? You've done my work for me! I might be able to get this accepted into the April meeting of the committee that makes decisions about whether or not we go forward with the case to a hearing. Could you fax me a copy?"

"Well, there's a problem with these records. They show all the doctors I've seen for two years before Blackwood, not just him."

"Usually on records like this the names of all the other doctors are blacked out with magic marker."

That's when I began to learn a great deal about photocopying.

Judith instructed, "Black out everything. They'll hold it up to the light and try very hard to read what's there. You may need to photocopy it, black it out, and then photocopy it again. Be very meticulous."

A few days later I stood once again in the foyer of the College of Physicians and Surgeons and immediately liked the intelligent look of the investigator on the case. I handed Judith nineteen pages of official health records listing the visits Blackwood had been paid for, including the brief hugs. Unbelievable. In my Letter of Complaint one of my sections was titled, "He Saw Me Excessively."

"Here's nineteen pages of 'He Saw me Excessively.'"

"I guess that proves it," Judith said without cracking a smile as she took the envelope.

So, she had a sense of humour.

During my next phone call with the investigator I learned that the College was going forward with my case quickly: my Letter of Complaint and records were going to the Complaints Committee that month. I also learned that Judith wanted to have the originals of the letters he wrote to me and all other things that could possibly be used as evidence. I had mentioned to her that I had calendars of my dates with him after the therapy.

Judith said, "Those are gold. Doctors are *never* allowed to see their therapy patients socially."

"He told me it was okay after six months." Then I said, "I have a letter asking me to have a relationship with him after the office relationship was over."

Judith made an effort to keep the excitement out of her voice. "I need the original, in case we have to send his handwriting to forensics."

I balked at that. "I may need the originals for the civil case; the evidence will have to be shared. What system do you have in place for this?"

"The College doesn't share."

"Oh." Except with the defence, I thought.

"We'll use everything you have. Too bad victims don't know ahead of time that they're going to report the doctor. It's basically their word against the doctor's. Sometimes a victim can get the doctor on tape admitting everything. Those cases are a lot easier."

"No tape," I said gloomily.

"Well, if you ever hear of someone who thinks they're being abused, tell them to get a tape of the doctor saying something incriminating. Tell them they can put a cheap tape recorder in their purse. Or use their cell phone to get a photo."

I changed the subject. "I'm worried about my personal safety. I constantly run into him in my neighbourhood. I mean, it figures, right, because we live in the same part of Toronto, my husband and I both see him a lot."

"I'll get a statement from your husband," said Judith.

My mind tilted a bit. I hadn't told Richard yet.

"He shows up on my running route. And when I walk the dog. I find it all very unnerving. He terrifies me."

"Change the locks on your doors."

That night my body seemed to float in fragments around me. Being interviewed by the College about what happened in Blackwood's office would be impossible. I knew I would faint. I had to see Maggie.

Was I doing the right thing? The civil suit, if there was going to be one, upset me as well. I had lost my career because of Blackwood and my family was now in terrible debt. I felt robbed and wanted my money back. Would they take my case knowing I was poor? Exactly why was I suing Blackwood anyway?

During my first meeting with my civil lawyers Jeff Duffy had said, "Getting money is one way of getting justice." I was so astounded by the idea of justice I couldn't hear anything else Duffy said. How could I possibly get back what I had lost? I wondered what a decade from the prime of a career was worth. Or not being present for my children. Almost losing my marriage? Losing my mind? Losing my religion? I had been completely robbed of who I used to be. I would have to say that it's impossible to put a price tag on these losses. For losses like these, there is no justice.

My mind leapt from the civil suit back to the College hearing. How did I feel about the possibility of a doctor losing his license to practice medicine? Was I rubbing my hands in joy? No, it felt awful. I knew Blackwood's kids, his ex-wife, some of his friends. We lived in the same neighbourhood. But if his license had been so important to him he would have stuck to the rules.

And he knew the College's rules. That's why it was negotiated that *I* would place *his* fingertips on myself so that I wouldn't be able to report him. He could then argue that I made him do it. Since when does a patient make a doctor do anything?

And was justice really just civilized revenge?

Maggie stopped moving her fingers and looked at me. "What's there now?" Maggie and I were preparing for my interview with the College investigator.

"I feel like I'm in an airplane and I can't land because the runway has disappeared. Everything is vibrating and the skin has melted off my bones as I hurtle through space. I keep trying to land but the ground is a mirage. I feel myself shimmering, it's as if my bones are flying apart. Skin is helpful, Maggie, it holds bones together. My brain simply refuses to remember being in his office."

Maggie asked, "Where do you feel it in your body?"

I laughed ruefully, "I don't have a body. That's why I'm here." I looked at Maggie deadpan, "Or not."

Maggie laughed and then waited for me to speak.

I somehow found some courage. "I am going to try to visualize being in his office. Will anything bad happen?"

"Like what?"

I didn't really know. Maybe I thought I would die. It felt like that.

I took a calming breath. "Okay, I'm ready. If I die, well, I'll have a good reason not to be at my Monday meeting with the investigator." I laughed at myself. "It all feels so familiar, this fear."

"That's why you got abused by him in the first place, because you were abused as a child. You had no idea that you were being abused as an adult. It was familiar, it was what you knew."

Maggie started to move her fingers back and forth in front of my eyes while I tried again to place myself in Blackwood's office. I started to cry but kept going. My mind was sorting the dark black blur of memories into visible detail: how he smelled; how his touch felt; how I felt.

In my mind I relived the events where Blackwood stood behind me and pressed his body against me. Most of the times when he did this, he had an erection. He would wrap his arms loosely around me while I imagined I was being sexually attacked. I saw myself turning in his arms towards him, burying my face in his chest, and imagining being rescued by him. I visualized him fighting off my attacker. We had done this same rape routine so many times.

Maggie stopped moving her fingers. "What's there now?"

"It was terrifying. And now I know why. In his office, during a rape scene, I imagined that I was being sexually attacked and I was, only by Blackwood. I will never forgive him for telling me my father had abused me. The nightmare began because I turned to an attacker in my actual reality to be saved from an attacker that he created in my mind."

Maggie was following what I was saying. "This gave you a sense of very grave danger. You had been terrified in his office, but you didn't know why. You trusted your doctor to keep you safe."

"You get it," I was so relieved that Maggie understood. "I could have killed myself because of the tormenting fear. As it was, I only went crazy. He drove me crazy."

"Yes, he did."

Maggie leaned forward and resumed the EMDR therapy. Ever so slowly I climbed up through the murky waters of the well of my guilt and eventually latched onto the elusive idea that what happened to me might not be my fault.

"Take a breath in and let it out," Maggie said. "What's there now?"

I choked out the words. Tears flowed as the memories flashed in rapid fire on the screen inside my eyes. "I remember it all: the feel of the berber carpet under my bare legs; the way the light slid through the slats in the venetian blinds as I looked up from the floor; the ivory phone covered in dirty fingerprints; the grimy wood grain on the teak desk; the sound of the chipped drawer opening as David took out my special cloth to put on the pillow on the floor; the sound of his heart beating while he hugged me; his hot breath on the back of my neck as he pressed his erection against me and pretended to be my father raping me; the weird muscle in his bum. I remember it all, vividly. It's a nightmare."

Maggie's fingers again moved back and forth in front of my eyes until the fear in my body finally evaporated.

Now I could be interviewed.

CHAPTER 22

THE CIVIL LAWSUIT NEEDED preparation as well. I went down to my basement and opened up my filing cabinet for the first time in years. Lawsuits are about money, and I needed to prove my income for the five years prior to my first appointment with Blackwood.

As I was sneezing my way through all the dusty files I came across a single page of linen bond—the off-white textured paper I used for my resume—which was a concise summary of all my publications: thirty-six produced plays; nineteen books; thousands of publications in papers all across the country with my syndicated children's column; cover stories; educational software design; video scripts; a magazine for teachers; weekly submissions for one of Toronto's daily papers. My hand stroked the page fondly; how I had enjoyed writing for children for twenty years. And then it had all shuddered to a stop. All my dedication to children's literacy had evaporated into hundreds of shitty poems to Blackwood.

With tears running down my cheeks, I gathered up the files and stuffed them back into the metal drawer.

It clanged shut.

That night I wrote about shutting the filing cabinet and it sounding like I was shoving a dead body into the fridge at the morgue.

"He destroyed my reason for being. *Why* I wrote."

Barbara asked, "What did you feel when you read that summary of your work?"

"So sad. So very sad." I began to cry again. "I was a children's writer, Barbara. I just wanted kids to laugh and love reading. Well, you know what? That man destroyed me."

Barbara was looking at me intently. "You still have talent, Kathy. You still write."

I didn't hear her. "All those crappy poems to Blackwood? I was just trying to survive."

"And you did. You're a good writer, Kathy."

Yes, but a really bad person.

The phone rang and the junior lawyer for my civil suit, Dylan, informed me that because I had no money they'd had to think very carefully about taking my case. And that the process was a fluid one. And that there might come a point in time when they would have to withdraw, depending on what arose.

"So you'll take it? Knowing I'm impecunious?"

"For now. As I said, this could change at any moment. But I need to talk to you about some costs. We'll need $5,000 up front."

"I can do that." Thank heavens for Ann! Then I listened to the lecture like a good child. They needed the money for photocopying. Photocopying seemed to be a major portion of legal proceedings. Lawyers needed lots and lots of paper. At the end of the call, I leapt and danced around my kitchen. The dog watched me and opened his furry lips into a cute little smile.

"I have a case, a case," I sang and danced as I wagged my finger at my dog, who wagged his tail back. "A nut case."

Two days later, at 9:31 am, there was a knock on the door. I opened it with what I hoped was confidence and invited the two people in.

"Hello, you'll remember me, Judith Harrison, and this is a social worker I work with, Nancy Scully."

I looked at Judith's outstretched hand and felt the blood drain from my body. I didn't touch hands. Hands were out. *Out out out.*

But I knew I had to be normal. Or appear to be. So I held out my hand and shook Judith's. Relief flooded through me, I couldn't feel a thing! Ha ha, I was numb. Good trick.

"Hi. Come in. Let me take your coats."

Judith turned on a tape recorder and asked me questions. I was so glad I had been to Maggie the week before; their very first set of questions was about Blackwood's office. Judith kept harping about his window. What on earth could be so interesting about a window? Yes, he had one. It had a blind. So what?

"Describe the window to me."

"Well, it had square panes, was painted white, was often open, there was a blind, it was usually down, but then it was broken and David kept it up. The window I mean." No one laughed. I inwardly sighed.

"What could you see out of the window?"

"A brick wall."

"You couldn't see another window? Pipes? Anything?"

"I saw bricks."

What on earth could she be getting at? What was so important about a ratty old window? And then Judith moved on to the flooring.

"Do you remember what type of flooring was in his office?"

I prayed she wasn't going to go on about the carpet like she had the window and tried to cut her off at the pass. "It was gray, nubbly carpet, short loop. Berber. Grimy, even though he'd replaced the previous brown." That seemed to satisfy her because she went on to another feature of his office: the lighting.

Now this line of questioning I felt was relevant: Blackwood always turned out the light when I walked into his office.

"Describe the lighting to me."

"There was an overhead fan light."

"What's that?"

Judith didn't know? I looked closely at her face. No, she really didn't know. "It's like an airplane propeller that spins around and at the center of the propeller is a light."

"How do you turn it off?"

"With a switch, beside the door." I remembered him slinking past me on silent feet to turn off the light. I remembered him saying, "You can call me partner" and me thinking, "said the spider to the fly."

"What happens to the fan?"

"It stops."

"Were there any other lights?"

"Yes, one over the examining table."

My mind skittled back to him looking up my vagina because I had a stomach ache. Bastard.

For five gruelling hours they sat at my dining room table, asking me questions, listening to me read my Letter of Complaint, taping me. Every fifteen minutes Judith ejected a used up tape and snapped in a new one. She seemed to be constantly unwrapping, flipping, and shoving them into the recorder. I wanted to shriek that she could buy longer tapes at Wal-mart.

During one of the five-minute breaks, Judith went upstairs to go to the bathroom. But she didn't come down. What was she doing? I listened carefully. Opening my cupboards? Yes, I was sure I heard the soft slide of a drawer. What would Judith think about the incriminating bottle of Tums? The ibuprofen? She finally came downstairs, looking innocent.

I asked the investigators what they thought about some statistics I got off the Internet. "I found an article that said fifty percent of women who go for therapy from a general practitioner in private practice ended up being sexually abused by the doctor."

Judith said, "Is that all?"

After they left, I put on my track shoes and ran and ran.

I was still puffing by the time the kids got home from school.

A month later Judith called. "We're going to Blackwood's office in a few days to seize your chart. Our visit will be unannounced."

Oh no. I wanted to be as far away from him as possible when Judith had this little foray. "I think I'll go to Nova Scotia. I'll stay with a friend."

"Give me your number there; I'll call right after we visit Blackwood."

Three days later Judith called. I was sitting in my friend Diane's kitchen when the phone rang. I jumped, my heart leaping erratically in my chest.

"Hello? Kathy?"

"Hi, Judith. How did it go?" My heart somersaulted, missing a beat. A heart attack?

"I gave him your Letter of Complaint to read and he admitted it was true. Not all of it, but most of it."

Fear started blistering my skin as I imagined Blackwood reading my letter and saying it was true. "It's *all* true, Judith. What did he say?" My voice was tinny.

"He said he watched you masturbate, but that it happened just once. That he knew it was inappropriate."

I snorted.

"He admitted kissing you on College Street. He said he French kissed your cheek."

"It was so disgusting."

"He also said he used a 'healing hand' and that he impersonated your father."

The rape rituals scudded across my mind. "What else?"

"He admitted he negotiated contracts. That he held you like a child while he leaned his back against his examination table. I think he'll fold, Kathy. He's admitted it."

"No he won't, you don't know him. He won't take responsibility for his actions. You don't know what he's like."

"What I do know I don't like. He gives me the creeps. I'll never forget his handshake. Like he's evil or something."

"I know." Unfortunately I knew his hands only too well.

"It sounds like encouragement to me, and that's important. Because encouraging you to masturbate will definitely cost him his license, that's a for sure. The other things? Well, he might get off."

"He touched my clitoris. I know he'll lose his license for doing that. Besides, he encouraged me to masturbate all right. But it's still my fault."

Judith audibly sighed. "No, it's not, Kathy."

I said nothing.

"The office was just as you described it."

So, who was being investigated? Me or the doctor?

"Judith, he knew what he was doing was wrong. He sneered, 'I'll only get my wrists slapped.'"

"Oh, he'll get more than that, believe me."

But my frustration flared. "What is this? He admitted it. And yet he can still go to work and touch other women? In any other industry the guy would be dismissed from his duties until the results of the investigation were known. But not doctors, oh no. The very people who have unrestricted access to women's bodies can continue accessing them, because, after all, they are gods saving people's lives."

"Don't worry, Kathy. I think he'll fold."

We said goodbye and I watched the fog roll across the field. I whispered into the empty room, "He's not going to fold. Not Mr. Liar, Liar, pants on fire. No way."

Late that night I was sitting in the kitchen by myself, listening to the sea sighing in the distance and the fire crackling in the woodstove. Diane had gone to bed long ago. I stared at the black pane of glass in the kitchen window, knowing that outside there was mist swirling around in the fields. I was on my fifth beer. I was drunk.

Every now and then I shook my head. He shouldn't have admitted it. I muttered, "What an asshole." Unbelievable that he could be so stupid to admit it. I called him an asshole over and over again. "They're all assholes," I whispered. And then I began to cry and rock back and forth, trying to keep warm by the woodstove.

Back in Ontario, I called Judith at the College. "Did you get his Letter of Defence yet?"

"He's asked for another extension."

"Another? What's going on? He's on holiday?"

Judith didn't answer. So he was.

"I see," I fumed and hung up, furious.

So much for doctors obeying the mandated response time of thirty days as set out in the *Regulated Health Professions Act*. I had looked it up. He'd now taken almost two months to reply!

Ann was right. That act was useless.

Months later, I read the eight pages of his Letter of Defence. Wasn't sexual from his perspective! A single time where I self-stimulated! Difficult patient! Didn't he know how bad it would look lying to the College, his ruling body?

He was such a liar.

I sat at the dirty pub table eating a toasted western with Ann and stealing her fries. "He'll get off you know. He lies. He's even lied in his Letter of Defence to the College. But people believe doctors. They're like gods. He'll win. Why should I bother doing this?"

Ann snarled, "You were a victim. A victim. Grow up and expose the jerk."

"What do you mean I was a victim?"

Ann sighed loudly, as if I were a total idiot. "A victim is a person who is in the wrong place at the wrong time."

"But don't they ask for it?"

Ann's whole face shook with rage and indignation. She spluttered, blowing discarded sugar packets across the table. "No." The word whistled out of her like steam escaping from a pressure cooker. "You were a *victim*. You were in the wrong place at the wrong time. Period.

Wrong place, wrong time. That's *all*." She took a long drink of her spiked coffee and banged it down on the table.

"So, victims are innocent." I mulled over this novel idea. "A victim is simply a person who is in the wrong place at the wrong time. Maybe one day I'll write a book about all this. And Ann, that line's going in."

"Stop eating my fries."

CHAPTER 23

THE COLLEGE INVESTIGATOR, JUDITH, and I had just finished going over the transcript of my taped interview. I brushed some breakfast crumbs off the table. Judith was running her fingers through her hair, making it flop lazily on her shoulders.

"How are you doing with all this, Kathy?"

"Okay, I guess. Not really. You know Judith, if there were a before and after shot of me seeing the doctor, I think you'd assume you were looking at an after shot, because I seem pretty okay now. But the after shot is a picture of nothing. Of TV snow. You know when the cable cuts out?"

"When it goes all gray and sounds like static?"

"That would be a pretty good picture of who I was after seeing that doctor. I had ceased to exist as a human being. I was hissing in nothingness."

"At some point we will need a Victim Impact Statement from you." Judith was watching me intently.

"How on earth can I tell a group of people that I suddenly disappeared from the face of the earth because my power had been yanked from the wall of faith and I became nothing at all but a blank screen of vibrating TV snow? They'll think I'm cuckoo."

Judith pushed her chair away from the table and said, "Don't worry Kathy, you'll be fine."

I was far from fine. I couldn't even sit in front of a lake without thinking of death. Waves were the colour of gun metal and marched tirelessly towards me, chanting, "We are dead and you are dead, we are dead and you are dead." All I could think of was guns coming to shoot me and how frightened I was of the lake. Not because it was coming to kill me, but because it was dead. How could a dead thing shoot me?

But I knew, because the lake was dead, that my greatest loss was my god from the landscape. As I sat by the lake this knowledge made me suicidal; I had lost the core of my being. And although years had passed since Blackwood had robbed me of this essential foundation of my soul, I still had not killed myself. Why bother, I thought as I watched the waves aiming their gray waves at me. I was already dead.

Richard worked hard at work and earned a bonus trip to the Wasatch Mountain Range, to Sundance, where Robert Redford had built a beautiful resort. "You seem so down, Sky, I wish you'd tell me why. Let's go on this trip and have some fun."

"Sure honey. Thanks. We'll have fun." Barrel of laughs.

As I looked off my chalet balcony all I could see were black dry mountains full of dust, blocking out light, freedom and air. Every morning Richard would fling the shutters open and exclaim, "Beautiful!"

He had worked so hard to earn this trip for us, so I, lying on the couch with my head back and pinching the base of my nose to stop a nosebleed from the altitude, did my best to be cheerful. "Yes sweetie, fabulous."

I had to tell Richard about Blackwood. I had to.

Richard was sitting in a Muskoka chair at the cottage, reading a car magazine. I could see him from the kitchen window. *Now or never,* I thought. I put the kettle on, made him a cup of tea, grabbed some cookies, and sat down beside him.

"Thanks sweetie," he said as he took the cup and small plate of cookies. "How did you know I was gasping for a cup of tea?"

"That's okay, hon. Listen, there's something I have to tell you." I eased myself into a chair beside him and stared at the waves on the lake. "Something serious."

"Shoot."

I winced at his choice of words.

"Well, you remember Dr. Blackwood?"

Richard nodded, his mouth full.

"He, um, he, ah-h-h, he sexually abused me and I've reported him to the College of Physicians and Surgeons."

Richard went very still. I wanted to brush away the cookie crumb from the corner of his mouth. Somewhere a crow cawed.

"So, now you know." I turned away and looked straight ahead. Sunlight danced on the lake between the trees. The drone of a lawnmower hummed in the distance.

"Don't report him Sky."

"I already have. Past tense. It's done. I had to Richard. He drove me crazy. He can't do what he did to me to other women. Some would die. I almost did. Besides, it's a terrible problem. Doctors abuse women all the time. It's worse than priests, Richard. Fifty percent of women who go to their GP for therapy end up being sexually assaulted."

"It's your word against his. You have no proof. Back out."

"I won't. It's done. I've started a lawsuit as well."

Richard processed the information while drinking his tea. I pretended I was trying to get a tan and forced my arms to look relaxed on the wide arms of the Muskoka chair. I was so frightened he'd be really, really angry. I heard his cup go down on the plate. It wasn't a slam.

"Well," Richard stood up, "haven't you been a busy little bee. Let's go for a paddle, honey. It's a perfect dog day."

I looked at him and said, "Woof." It was our in-joke. Everything would be okay.

As we paddled along Richard asked me, "Did you have sex with him?"

"Oh, no honey, I couldn't do that."

"But you had that fight about the note. I thought you loved him."

The sentence drifted in the air as we paddled in unison. His pain throbbed just slightly above the canoe. How could I possibly explain what had happened to me?

"I didn't love him, Richard. I had a fiercely strong emotion for him and I had to label it 'love.' Anything else would be unimaginable. It's how I kept myself safe from the knowledge that I was being abused. My world would have come to an end if I had to acknowledge what I knew deep down, before I was ready. He touched me sexually all over to rewire me. He acted out raping me, Richard. He told me my father abused me. Then he told me to call him 'Daddy' while he encouraged me to masturbate for him. It was terrifying. I *had* to believe he loved me. I *had* to believe I loved him."

I watched the water swirl around my paddle while I waited for Richard to reply. Everything was so quiet. I could hear some ducks take off across the bay. The breeze rustled in the bull rushes.

Richard stuck his paddle in. "Fucking bastard."

I was a mess. Toward the end of the summer I drove, once again, with my son and two of his friends to my lovely shack by the sea in Nova Scotia. I stopped at the highway motel I always stopped at and after they were asleep, sat on a plastic chair outside the motel room and listened to the night sounds. I heard the far-off humming from the highway, the low buzz of air conditioners, and a punctuating hoot of laughter from the patio bar around the corner of the parking lot. I took a swig of beer. Then I tilted way back on the chair and looked up at the moon.

I felt as if I had been blasted from a cannon in outer space and was falling towards earth. On my way down I encountered a sound barrier. This was where my cries met the dark mesh of night, the barrier trapping and sifting my pain from the air. As I looked up I wondered if all those trapped screams in the layers of sky would escape and slice through the atmosphere like broken bits of glass into my mouth.

Suddenly a sheet of heat lightning lit up the night. For a second the whole universe was illuminated by a flash of blue light. The shining clarity of everything around me was startling. I burst out laughing.

I had seen the light! Ha ha. And there was nothing there!

There were no screams trapped behind a sound barrier. There was no barrier. There was no sound at all. I wondered if my faith had been restored as I sat in my plastic chair and listened to the cacophony of peace.

Someone burped at the outdoor bar. I laughed and laughed.

After the summer was over, Judith arrived at my door with a huge rolling briefcase stuffed with papers, including, I knew, the buff-coloured file, my therapy chart, that Blackwood had written in to record our sessions.

"Soon you're going to need a Sherpa guide to carry all the paper you have for this case," I laughed. Judith didn't. This was serious business.

"Just remember what I told you yesterday: don't get angry."

I sighed as I took Judith's jacket. "I am nowhere near angry."

Judith sat at my dining room table and pulled out my therapy chart from her briefcase.

I flicked the file folder open. "I don't understand these dates." I was flipping through the pages while my heart hammered in my ribs.

"They start from the last time you saw the doctor and move back into time."

"Oh great," I sighed, "just what a dyslexic needs."

I read with embarrassed horror the gushing thank you letter I had written to Blackwood. But the two poems I had so perfectly folded weren't in the file. "Already I see something missing: this letter came with two poems. There was a great one with a line in it about his hands melting a block of ice, in other words, me, as he touched me and how the water foamed pink with his blood. It just isn't here."

"Don't get angry," said Judith quickly.

I raised my eyebrows at her. Judith's head was down as she whipped through pages, feverishly making big red squares around blocks of his handwriting. I had never seen her so focused. Judith's eyes moved back and forth across the lines of Blackwood's tiny writing. Every now and then she'd look up, full of amazement and whisper unbelievingly to me, "It's in the box."

David, in his tight little handwriting, had written down almost everything he had done to me! He had recorded the rewiring, the rapes, the hugs, the masturbating, everything! I had irrefutable proof!

The investigator was circling madly. There was a lot "in the box." And there were a lot of boxes. And then abruptly she stopped, shut the file, and said, "That's enough."

I had completely detached myself from where I was; Judith's words resonated in my mind as if they were coming from far away. "I told you he did it."

I struggled with staying in reality. My insides were trembling. He did it. I hadn't made it up. My memory was accurate. Oh Christ. Something inside me wailed.

"This file is a godsend," trumpeted Judith. "Look," she said as she re-opened the file. "Here it is in black and white; you lay on the floor, he sat at your head, the two of you locked eyes, and you told him sexual fantasies while you 'self- stimulated.'" She pointed at the passage in the chart with her finger.

"Imagine him writing it down," I croaked. "What an asshole."

Judith looked at me and frowned. She didn't like swearing.

"Sorry." My stomach was churning. "I don't know if I can go through with this, Judith. He's obviously very sick. He should know to hide what he did. He needs a great deal of help."

"Do you think a person who is lacking in judgment to this extent should be practicing medicine?"

"Oh." My wave of compassion petered out.

"We're stopping. Your neck is bright red, Kathy. That's a sign of severe distress."

"Guess I better buy myself a turtleneck for the hearing."

She shook her head and tapped the file. "And now what do you think the chances are of Blackwood folding?"

"Still nil."

Judith raised her eyebrows. I spread my hands and shrugged.

I thought for a minute. "Why wasn't this chart read months ago? When you first got it? It would have saved a lot of time and anguish. The proof is irrefutable."

"Don't worry, he'll fold," Judith replied.

Why didn't she answer my question?

"No, he won't. The man has no moral integrity. He won't fold Judith because he doesn't believe he's done anything wrong."

"I'm going to get his file transcribed. I'm having trouble reading it."

"What? I don't. It's pretty legible."

"Put it this way: I don't believe what I'm reading. I'm also going to get an IO, an Independent Opinion from a psychiatrist that we use in situations like this."

Judith packed up her papers with staccato-like movements.

She handed me a copy of the file but she was very clear. "Under no circumstances are you to read this chart alone. Go over it with your EMDR therapist."

And soon I knew why. The minute Judith left the house, I got in my car and headed over to Blackwood's, yelling wildly, "You did it. It happened. You wrote it down. You told me you loved me. I believed you. Oh good, there's a blue car. Good, there's another. You did love me. Why didn't you love me?"

My cries echoed around and around in my car as I drove around and around his house.

That night I had nightmares about a lion eating my belly in a dark cave.

No way was I going to look at the file.

I sat in my office, staring at my hands, not being able to write. Finally I wrote at the top of the page, "Under My Skin" and began to mutter.

"My hands touched David like they've never touched anyone before. That's why I've cut them off. And now the words are stockpiling at my wrists. Maybe they'll multiply and take over my whole body. Then my bones and blood will be writhing with them like maggots. One day there'll be so many of them that the awful disgusting words will seep out like pus and I will finally have to describe how I touched him."

I ripped up the page.

Judith called me and said, "The psychiatrist we used to give an opinion on your chart said it was the worst case of sexual abuse he's ever seen. We've been using this psychiatrist for years for Independent Opinions and his reputation is impeccable. Blackwood will be slapped with an Order of Restrictions on his license to practice. He won't be able to do some things. How are you doing with this information, Kathy?"

The College certainly wasn't my friend. I was angry and spat, "Are you crazy? He shouldn't be practicing at all. Sexual abusers don't understand restrictions. That's the whole point. That's why they do what they do. Why doesn't the College understand that abusers have a fatal flaw? They have no boundaries? That they are morally sick?"

Judith ignored me. "The hearing will be within a few months. He has to make a living, and it's hard if he has restrictions."

"I haven't worked in years, Judith." I replied quietly.

The worst case the College shrink had ever seen? I lay down on my back in my office and listened to my EMDR relaxation tape. I wasn't crying, but tears kept rolling out of my eyes. They trickled down the sides of my cheeks and into my ears. I was dreadfully worried that the headphones would be damaged, that the foam ear cup would disintegrate into rubbery sawdust. And then I thought, "What if I get electrocuted?"

After surviving so much, I would be really pissed off if the newspaper headline said "Woman Killed by Walkman."

I ran every day. Three kilometres. No hills. On many days panic would topple peace and grip me so badly on my run that I felt I was on fire. I would race to Marion's. "I feel like my skin is burning off. It keeps burning off. I keep walking through fire."

Marion would hold me in her arms and stroke my hair. "It's okay, Sky. Shhh. It's okay. It's over. You're safe."

"But I feel like I'm walking through fire," I often wept.

"This too shall pass."

It did. I really was getting better.

CHAPTER 24

I STARTED TOYING WITH the idea of trusting Barbara. Maybe it was time to tell her more. "I've written a lot of poems called 'The Recovery Room'," I said as I held up a fistful and showed her. "In them I often have no legs. I chewed them off because they were in a trap and I had to get away. But then I couldn't get away because I had no legs."

I looked at her. "Win some, lose some."

Barbara didn't laugh.

"A lot of them are about dark air coming in under the recovery room door and poisoning me. And some are about a heart monitor beeping away, letting me know I am alive. Sometimes the doctor in the recovery room touches me and the recovery room turns into a cave. In this one," I held up a piece of paper, "the doorknob frightens me because it leads to outer space. I don't really know what they mean."

"I think the doctor mentioned in the poems is me," said Barbara, adjusting her jacket.

What? How could that be? How could I be writing all these poems and not know *that*? But of course they were about her. "There go the corners of the room."

I talked to Barbara about my fear of Blackwood. "I feel nothing but terror. It masks and jumbles up every other emotion. It confuses my thoughts. I feel as if I've been tossed into a volcano like a sacrificial virgin. I don't know why he had to do what he did. I feel like I'm hiding inside the volcano as it erupts and I'm pressing myself against the side, hiding from the lava, steam, heat, molten rock. I have disappeared into the focus of the effort of staying alive. But Barbara, the volcano is inside me. I have kept it alive inside myself at my very core. I know where I've been these whatever number of years."

I had utterly lost track of time.

Barbara looked up, tilted her head appraisingly, and wrote something down.

"I have spent so much time just surviving my constant feelings of fear that I haven't been able to feel anything else. I have no other emotions but fear. It's in all my poems. Do you think I'm a good writer?"

"Yes. I've told you that before. Do you?"

"Yes I do. I feel good about my writing."

"What you're feeling is pride."

"Oh." I hugged this nugget of knowledge, this new emotion, to my chest.

After this, slowly but surely, I became aware of soft waves of various emotions floating around my heart. How I loved this, or hoped for that, or desired something. As the over-riding fear in me disappeared, I slowly became myself.

But should I trust my psychiatrist? She was a doctor, after all.

Just as I was beginning to stabilize, Blackwood began harassing me in my neighbourhood. He drove up and down my street and kept appearing in his car on my running route. He looked like a nightmarish cartoon, putt-putting along in his little blue car with an odd hat on his head. TV snow started eating at the corners of my mind again. I felt myself becoming unhinged and wobbled to Barbara.

"I see him and I get so frightened."

Barbara asked kindly, "What are you frightened of?"

I saw his face between my legs, his fangs glinting in the light coming from under the door and shadows flickering up his head. I was frightened he was going to eat me.

"I don't know." I couldn't speak the horrible truth.

"How do you feel when you see Dr. Blackwood in your neighbourhood?

I raced through my answer in a panic. "I feel like I have no value. Like I want to die. Like I am dead. That I have no dignity. That I am very frightened. That I am unsafe. That I want to kill myself."

"Prozac would help." She made a note.

What? Didn't the psychiatrist understand he frightened me? My breath came in sharp rasps. I was angry. And then I found my voice.

I spoke as calmly as I could. "Dr. Blackwood sexually assaulted me on a daily basis for over two and a half years. He terrifies me. Imagine being told to take Prozac. Here, take a little pill and your world will be safe?"

My anger escalated into fury. "I am being harassed. By a sexual offender. I don't need Prozac," I shouted, "I need the POLICE!"

No fucking way would I trust her. I grabbed my rumpled coat and pitched my body to the door. How unfair to find a voice and not be able to see straight.

I talked to Marion about Barbara's suggesting Prozac. "Seeing her is elective. Why should I see someone who disrespects my stand on chemicals in the body, who doesn't understand the impact of sexual assault?"

Marion replied, "Barbara has been very good for you. Look where you are, Sky. Did she *really* make a mistake? You told her you felt like killing yourself. You have to stop doing that, Sky. You're lucky she didn't call 911 right then and there and get the little men with the straitjackets to take you away, ha ha, to the loony bin."

"Oh," I said, somewhat deflated. "But I threaten to kill myself all the time. I never do and my psychiatrist, of all people, should know I won't kill myself because I am already dead. I told her that." I threw my head back and gulped some air.

"I understand, Sky. Barbara doesn't want you to suffer. She takes care of you. But you're not dead and you don't have to go to such extremes to make a point. Stop threatening with that. All you have to say is that it upsets you when you see him in your neighbourhood. Of course it does: he assaulted you."

Maybe I would trust Barbara.

Of course Barbara was upset. I said, "I understand that you just wanted me to feel better and I understand about your training. But I would never accept drugs. I'm sorry I said I felt like killing myself."

"I am on your side."

"I don't trust very well."

Barbara gave me one of her "you-don't-say" looks. I smiled ruefully.

In that moment I realized that Barbara mattered to me. The question was, did I matter to Barbara? Would I dare ask the question?

After Blackwood, I would have to find every ounce of my courage to ask. But I needed to know. What if Barbara pushed me? Shouted at me? Wind seemed to whirl around my ears as I took a deep breath.

"Do you care about me?"

"Of course I do."

I thought about that for a long, long time.

But my body was falling apart again. I had to keep going to the chiropractor because I just couldn't stand up straight. It was as if I had become permanently twisted in my effort to get away from Blackwood's penis pressed into my back. One day, after an appointment where I was somewhat straightened, I drove home thinking about how I now saw the earth.

My landscape was a crime scene. Nothing was left of my god but a crude chalk outline made with the dust of dry crumbling bones, startling white against the flat gray wall of my inner sky. The sharp outline showed where the essence of the land had been and scraped painfully against my mind. The land was so silent, so still, so empty, so very absent. Its holy spirit had simply disappeared, destroyed by Blackwood. And now my landscape was gone, leaving behind an empty chalk-drawn outline of bone against the sky. As I drove along I was utterly immersed in thought, thinking of how I'd lost my religion.

And then Mr. Nightmare Putt-putt showed up again, in his stupid blue car, just as I was almost home.

What did I do? Did I implode, evaporate into steam, turn into a volcano, have no value, want to kill myself, lose all my dignity, feel my body burning up? Not at all.

I said, "EEEEUUUUwww." Just like a girl does when she touches the slimy white underbelly of a fish.

So, who smelled now? I *was* getting better!

Marion and I were having lunch. "I'm thinking about writing a book."

Marion nibbled on a slice of cucumber. "About Blackwood? That's a big job."

"I don't know if I'll ever be able to write it." I took a bite of my sandwich. "Every time I sit down to write, even a little paragraph, my anxiety level soars through the roof. No matter how much yoga I do, how far I walk, how often I do my relaxation tape, I can't be calm when I sit in front my computer."

"Why not?"

"Just the usual: I'm stupid. Stupid, stupid, stupid." I sang.

Marion laughed. "You're not stupid, Sky."

"How stupid does one have to be to let a doctor run his hands over your body, time and time again."

"You were vulnerable, Sky. You were set up by your childhood. You had no way of figuring out it was abuse. You were his victim. He used you. He was bad. Not you. You're not stupid, you just didn't know."

"Sometimes his eyes glinted like Lynn's. I thought it was familiar. That it was okay. Ugh."

We ate our sandwiches in silence.

"You know he used his power as an aphrodisiac?" I piped up, as if this were a cheering thought.

"Yes, I know."

Well, I didn't have to actually write a whole book. Anything that struck me as unjust I would simply jot down, just in case.

Judith, the College investigator, called to say that Blackwood's Order of Restrictions was now specific: he wasn't allowed to do psychotherapy on individuals; he had to have a female nurse with him if he was examining a woman patient; and he had to post a sign in his waiting room saying what his restrictions were.

I got angry again. *Restrictions?*

I grit my teeth and called the lawyer that was representing the College against Blackwood. "Sexual abusers don't understand restrictions. That word does not exist in their vocabulary. That's why they do what they do. He wrote it down for heaven's sake. Take him right off the street! What is the College thinking?"

She said nothing.

My tirade lost some momentum. I knew I wouldn't win. "How big is the sign?"

"There are no guidelines."

"Oh great, so he can write it on the head of a pin so no one can read it. This is ridiculous. He's not going to post the sign. You know and I know he won't."

"He has to post the sign in his waiting room. It says so right on the Order at the bottom. He has to post the whole Order. Don't worry, he'll be monitored."

"By whom? Tell me that. Does the College actually employ monitors? People who run around and check if all the bad doctors are following the College's ridiculous Orders of Restrictions?"

"Well, no, but an investigator will check on him periodically."

"He's not going to post the sign. Not in his waiting room. I know it."

"As I said, I've made a note of your concern and will personally ensure that he will be monitored."

I snapped a goodbye and tried not to slam the phone down. Then I picked up the receiver and pounded it down hard. Twice. I was *so* frustrated.

I banged my fist on the kitchen counter, "Like fuck you will." I shook my head hard. "What fucking bullshit."

I yowled in my kitchen, "It's not the College *of* Physicians and Surgeons." My voice escalated an octave higher. "It's the College FOR Physicians and Surgeons." Then I shouted with frustration, "*For*, not *of!* Doesn't anyone know their goddamn fucking prepositions?"

The dog looked at me and seemed to be smiling. "Phew," I dusted my hands off. "That felt good." I checked the phone to see if I'd broken it. Good, a dial tone.

I shook my finger at my little dog. "That College is a fiasco. I'm going to do something. I don't know what. I'm so mad. I'm going to talk to Ann about this *crap*. It's *crap*. CRAP!"

The dog thought I had said "cat" and started racing around the kitchen, barking his head off.

CHAPTER 25

I REACHED ACROSS THE table and took another of Ann's french fries. I doused it with vinegar and swirled it through a glistening mound of ketchup. *Just one*, I thought, just one. And then I reached across the table for another. Couldn't let the ketchup go to waste, could I?

Between mouthfuls I said to Ann, "He's not going to post the sign you know. He doesn't operate within the boundaries of normal society. He's a sexual abuser. He lies. He rides his bike on the sidewalk. I just know he's not going to post the sign."

I took another fry. They were thick and delicious, crispy on the outside but soft and fluffy on the inside. Perfect.

"Imagine putting an Order of Restrictions on a sexual abuser. What assholes." I chewed another fry.

Ann's spoon clunked against the sides of her Irish coffee as she stirred in two packets of Equal. Ann was always watching what she ate. This was why the fries that came with her western sandwich were up for grabs. "What's the sign supposed to say? I know you told me once before, but refresh my memory."

I cast abandon to the wind, grabbed a handful of her fries and neatly lined them up in my leftover salad dressing. Great combo. I was on Weight Watchers and counted up the points as they lay like coffin nails in my salad bowl. If I ate them all I wouldn't be able to eat a thing for the rest of the week. Oh well. I reached for the salt and vinegar. "That he's supposed to post the sign in his waiting room outlining his restrictions."

Ann took a loud gulp of her coffee and scotch. "Which are…?"

"Well, that he can't do psychotherapy on individual women."

"But he can on couples?" Ann was incredulous.

I muttered, "Yes." I was so embarrassed by the College.

Ann's laughter blasted out of her mouth. "Jesus, how do they expect a man who abuses women to be of any help at all to couples?" Ann charged ahead, "Like, let's say a husband doesn't like what his wife is doing, is Blackwood going to say, 'Well, push her, that's what I do, just give her a shove.'"

The thought of Blackwood being allowed to give therapy to couples brought out the sarcasm in me. "Or if a husband is having trouble getting an erection, Blackwood would say, 'Watch her masturbate, my good man, works for me, no problem.'"

"What else does the Order say?"

"That he has to have a female nurse with him when he's with a female patient."

"And the College has assured you they will monitor him? Yeah right. By whom? It's up to you and me, Sky." Her spoon clanked as she stirred more Equal into her coffee.

"Ann..." I spoke as if disciplining a mischievous child, "What do you have up your sleeve?"

"I'm going to make an appointment to see him. For therapy. I'll make sure the sign is posted in his waiting room. That he has a nurse. If not, I'll call the media. What a great story."

I felt my stomach tremble. The last thing I wanted was to be named by a major Toronto daily. "I can't have my name in the paper."

"Don't worry. They have a policy never to print the names of victims of sexual assault."

"Oh. Okay then, do what you have to do." I was well aware that Ann always did what she wanted to do.

"I'm going to expose the fuckhead. Don't tell a soul you're in this with me. They'll be going on about conspiracy and revenge. This is all my idea."

"What idea?"

We both laughed. But in fact, it *was* all her idea.

"You know what else that stupid College did?"

"What?" Ann was ordering another of her spiked coffees.

"You know the Notice of Hearing that outlines the allegations against him?"

Ann nodded, leaning forward eagerly in her seat. She loved proof that the College was ridiculous.

"Although there is mention of various masturbating events, there is no mention of Blackwood masturbating Patient A. That would be me." I pointed at my chest. "And although I asked the prosecutor about this, she just gave me some waffle about how the Notice of Hearing can't contain everything, just some of the facts."

"Pretty important fact to leave out. Given it's the one main fact that will, without a doubt, cost him his license. Did he write down in his chart that he masturbated you?"

"Well, it's implicit in the rewiring sections. Him masturbating me was part of the rewiring." It wouldn't be enough proof. His lawyers would twist it around. But then I brightened up. "He wrote he touched my clitoris. It's in a list."

"And the allegations don't mention *that*? Something's up," Anne said, shaking her head. "They are not your friend. I keep telling you that. Repeat after me: the College is not your friend."

I obliged and chanted with Ann, "The College is not my friend."

"And I have to sign release forms for all my therapy charts for the civil suit. Dylan, my lawyer for the civil suit, has spoken."

"I told you they'd get everything. There is no privacy in Canada."

"They haven't got them yet. Shirley and Maggie and Barbara might refuse to hand them over. When I told Dylan this wouldn't happen in the States, you know what she said?"

"What?"

"'All very well, Kathryn, but this isn't the States.'"

Ann knocked back her coffee, slapped her credit card on the bill and gathered up her various bags. "Fuck 'em all."

Ann sank into the passenger seat of my car and wheezed. As she dug in her purse for her inhaler, beads of sweat dripped from her brow. The city was in the grip of a smothering heat wave so I had picked her up to drive her to Blackwood's office.

"How convenient, you're actually sick!"

"Yeah, maybe he'll give me some 'medicine.'" I had told Ann how he called his hugs "medicine." "We'll just see if the fuckhead even has a nurse."

I dropped Ann off at a corner near Blackwood's office and nervously watched her lumber away on the hot, dusty sidewalk. What Ann was about to do, put herself at the hands of a doctor who was a sexual abuser, was incredibly brave. I knew what Ann had been through and how much this exercise was going to cost her emotionally. She'd been abused by a priest *and* a doctor. No wonder she was so angry.

I backed my car under the shade of a maple and watched the shadows of leaves play along my windshield. I lowered my windows and turned off the ignition. As I leaned my head back against the headrest I imagined my friend in that dark office and inwardly quaked at the thought of Blackwood's hands on her. A soft summer breeze wafted across my face while I breathed deeply, trying not to panic, feeling that Ann would pick up on my distress. I don't know how much time had passed when I was jolted from my semi-doze. The door was yanked open and Ann fell into the car.

"No sign," she wheezed. "He didn't post it. Let's get out of here."

I threw the car into drive and the hot tires squealed as I wheeled around the corner.

"Did he have a nurse?"

"Yes," she panted. "But he wouldn't answer truthfully why she had to be there."

"Yeah, he's a liar." I raced the engine.

We went to our usual restaurant. Milk sprayed everywhere as Ann pulled foil off a little container with shaking hands. "Fucking things. Why don't they design a lid people can get off?" She dumped the milk into her double scotch coffee and stirred like a mad woman. Then she reached into her purse, grabbed her anti-anxiety pills and downed a couple, or more, with her spiked coffee.

I watched in horror. Drugs and drink? That's how my mother died!

"I can see why you fell in love with him. He seems very gentle and kind. That makes him all the more dangerous, doesn't it?" Ann's whole body shook as she took a deep gulp of her coffee.

I wasn't sure if her shudder was because of the insidious threat Blackwood posed to women, or if the scotch had grabbed Ann's tonsils on the way down and given them a hard shake.

"Oh, he's dangerous all right. His cruelty flows under the surface of his skin where no one can see it."

"Anyway, he hasn't posted the sign. I looked everywhere in his waiting room. It is not there."

"Of course not. So now what?"

"Now I call the media. The College has to be exposed for what they do. Protecting doctors, not the public. There's a reporter I trust. Would you be willing to talk to him?"

I stammered, "I guess so."

And then I stole all of Ann's fries. I'd given up on being thin.

Ann pulled out her cell phone and called a reporter, Don Pascussi, who said he'd go to Blackwood's office right away to check if he had posted the sign warning patients that he was operating under restrictions.

Twenty minutes later, Ann's cell phone chirped. She listened and then snapped it shut. "Pascussi says Blackwood posted the sign down a long hallway, at the bottom of a cluttered bulletin board, far away from the waiting room, near the bathroom. Well, *I* looked everywhere and didn't see it."

"You don't believe Pascussi?" I asked.

"Nope. I have to see that sign with my own eyes. If there is one, it's just been posted."

"So, um, what do you want to do now?"

"Go back and look for the sign." Ann spoke as if I was demented.

"Ah, won't that look kind of odd? You were just there."

"Well, I forgot my cell phone, didn't I?"

"Oh, cell phone. Of course. Good idea."

"I'll ask the receptionist if anyone turned it in and then go down the hall pretending to look for my phone in the bathroom."

The two of us ate in companionable silence until Ann noticed her fries were gone. "Hey! I thought you were on Weight Watchers."

"Oops..." I batted my eyelashes and tried to look innocent.

"Ha ha. Listen, I'm going to take my tape recorder. I'm going to get little miss curly top receptionist to speak right into it. What's her name again?"

"Lydia."

"Okay Lydia, here we come."

The heat wave still lay across the city like a heavy blanket while Ann and I, once again, drove up Bathurst Street to Blackwood's office. Ann was trying to get her small pocket-sized tape recorder to work reliably and kept clicking it on and off while swearing at it. A couple of times I grabbed the recorder and said, "Here, this is how it works."

Ann grabbed it back and said, "I'll do it my way, fuck you very much."

The heat was making us crabby.

Finally we arrived at the corner near Blackwood's and again I watched Ann lope to his office. I parked under the maple, lay back and dozed. I felt like I was on a stake-out. Suddenly between my half-shut lids, I saw Blackwood. He was just fifty yards from me, riding his bike on the sidewalk, heading south against northbound traffic. My heart raced and the blood drained out of my body. A chaotic combination of despair, anger, and hope flared in my heart as I watched the sun glint off his shiny helmet. Like a thousand prisms, rainbow spikes flashed between my eyelashes. And then he was gone.

I shut my eyes completely and waited for my heart to stop pounding. I'd make a lousy detective. No way would I be able to give chase on Gumby legs.

And then Ann huffed into view. She was scurrying around the corner toward my car, holding the silver tape recorder in the palms of her hands in front of her as if it were an offering to the gods.

She dumped her damp body into the passenger seat, "You won't believe what she said. I've got it right here on tape." She tapped the recorder hard with her jagged fingernail. "Quick, let's get to the restaurant."

Lydia's nasal whine grated out of the tiny recorder on the table in front of us. She was justifying why Blackwood hadn't posted the sign in his waiting room for everyone to see. "He'd never do what he's accused of. He's a good doctor. There are a lot of crazies out there."

Ann wheezed, "It was right on his Order of Restrictions that he was to post the sign in his waiting room. The sign was where Pascussi said it was, in the hall by the bathroom. But it didn't say Blackwood had to post it in his waiting room. He must have taken a pair of scissors and cut that part off. What a perv."

Later that day I was on the phone with the reporter, Don Pascussi. Pascussi sounded pissed off because he'd wasted his time on what turned out to be a false lead for a story. "I went and checked myself. Ann told me he hadn't posted the sign. He did, just not where people could see it. It's in a hallway at the bottom of a notice board filled with articles and jokes."

I laughed. "That's so Blackwood. Putting it in a hallway was violating the Order. But he cut off the part that stipulated it be in the waiting room. Bends the rules to suit himself. He didn't want his patients to see the sign, so he hid it. He's a menace. He should be suspended pending the results of a hearing. The evidence is overwhelming."

"What evidence?"

"He wrote it down. Didn't you know?"

"What do you mean? Wrote what down?" Don Pascussi's voice was slightly raised, as if on the scent of something big just around the corner.

"In his chart, his therapy file on me. He wrote down everything he did to me."

"You're kidding, right?"

"No. Right there in black and white it says in a list all the parts of me he touched, including my clitoris. Stuff like that. That he watched me masturbate."

"I don't believe it. Would you let me see the chart?"

By now I knew that my chart was going to be made public anyway. "Okay. I will. Other things will soon be public as well, like his Letter of Defence to the College. In it he contradicts things that are in his chart. For example he says to the College that I self-stimulated just one time, but his chart reflects many times. Like he thinks people can't connect the dots? He's a liar."

"I'd like to interview you."

Don Pascussi wrote for the same paper that I used to write for, long ago. As I entered the familiar building, emotion welled up inside me. I couldn't do my job as a children's writer for that newspaper because of Blackwood. I'd give the reporter what he needed. Fuck the College. They were more than useless.

Throughout the interview I kept flying in and out of reality. Here, not here. Here, not here. I wished I could stay focused and in my body. I breathed deeply and tried to sound intelligent, but I could feel nervous sweat making my legs stick to the plastic cover on the cafeteria bench. I slid my files across the table towards Pascussi. He read each page quickly, jumped up, and left. I could see him in another room, through the glass, photocopying like a maniac.

When he returned he asked, "The chart mentions love poems. Were you in love with him? I mean, how could that be? He was an abuser."

I was completely frazzled. "I don't know what to say about that."

"Why don't you think about it? I have to talk to my editor for a minute."

As soon as Pascussi charged up a stairwell, I blundered to a hallway and called Ann on my cell. I whispered loudly, "He's asked me something important. I'm not sure what. Abuse? Love? Maybe if I were in love with Blackwood. I think. I don't know. I'm dissociating. He asked me something. What was it?"

"Calm down. Take a deep breath." Ann spoke slowly, dragging out the words so I could hear them.

"He asked me a question about love and abuse. Those two words were in the question. What do I say?"

"Say that abuse has nothing to do with love and everything to do with power. You were in his power. He abused his power. His power was his aphrodisiac."

"Phew, thanks, good one."

Gratefully I snapped the phone shut and hurried back to my vinyl seat before Don returned. I pretended to be writing nonchalantly in my notebook and acted as if I were in possession of all my faculties as he slid into the booth. I said, "In answer to your question, yes, Blackwood is a sexual abuser. What sexual abusers do is use their power over someone as their aphrodisiac. Abuse has nothing to do with love. It is about power. Power over a person. I was spellbound in his power. Power can get masked as love."

Pascussi wrote it all down and I hoped it made a good quote. I wished I'd said that extreme fear is such a strong emotion that people who have been abused often interpret it as love so they don't have to face the reality of what's happening to them. Or that I had been abused as a child and didn't know I was being abused by the doctor. Whatever. I did the best I could, considering.

I could see Emma and Jamie sunbathing on the dock through the cottage window. Margaret was sitting in the shade, reading an Archie comic. Every now and then one of them would lazily plop into the water to cool off. It was so much easier now, I thought, now that they could all swim and I didn't have to watch them like a hawk. While they were all down at the water and I had the cottage to myself, I decided to make some phone calls. Pascussi's article had hit the Saturday paper and there was bound to be some reaction.

I called an old friend from high school, one of the three Marys I used to hang out with. I talked to the Mary's every now and then and I'd been thinking about them lately. It was time to connect. "Did you read the article in today's paper?"

"It was pretty explicit, Kath."

I heard the old nickname and was transported back thirty-some odd years, remembering when the Marys and I stood on the street corner and gabbed about everything school girls talk about.

"Well, it *is* a newspaper article, written by a journalist. Of course it is."

"I don't really want to know. I can't help you. "

What was this? I didn't need help. Not now. "Okay, so we won't talk about it."

But I knew from that very short telephone exchange that my thirty-five year old friendship had taken a beating and probably wouldn't survive. I was not interested in having relationships with people who couldn't face reality. I hung up the phone, saddened and sorely disappointed in Mary, but still somewhat hopeful the relationship would continue. Time would tell. Barbara and Maggie had both told me I would lose friends. Please not one of the Marys, I thought. Not one of my oldest friends. I didn't have the heart to call the other two Marys.

Richard had to work that Saturday, but when he arrived at the cottage later that night I could tell by the stiff way he hugged me that he was very upset. He pulled the Saturday paper out of his gym bag and threw it onto the coffee table.

"There. Happy?"

"I'm sorry Richard. But the College wasn't doing anything. Women are in danger."

"Keep this stuff away from the family. That's all I ask. "

I hid the newspaper in the bottom of the recycling bin.

CHAPTER 26

A S THE SUMMER HEAT permeated Ontario, I decided it was time to round up some kids and head out to my little house in Nova Scotia. Emma and Margaret had gone off to camp, so it was just Jamie and two of his friends. Right before I left, I stuffed the transcribed copy of Blackwood's chart into my briefcase. Although Maggie and I had gone over the chart together, I would have to know it inside and out before the College hearing. After driving for two days straight, we finally arrived. Gear was unpacked, dead flies were vacuumed, and food was put away. The boys made their beds in the shed, ate dinner, and then went outside to throw rocks at a metal sign. I sat at the rickety kitchen table, making a list of what I needed in town. Through the plinks of pebbles hitting the sign, I could hear the ocean sighing in the background and a lobster fishing boat chugging out of the harbour. After the dinner dishes were done and Jamie and his friends were giggling in the shed before they went to sleep, I curled my feet under me on the couch and took out the photocopy of Blackwood's chart from my nylon briefcase. Tossing the briefcase onto the couch beside me, I smoothed my hand over the first page.

For the first time I read the first thirty pages without Maggie. The past rose up from the dark recesses of my heart and hammered on the inside of my skull. I felt like I would shatter under the pressure of the terrifying memories. I started to gasp for air and my whole body began to tingle. TV snow hissed in my ears. I drank beer after beer, one after another, trying to drown the pictures in my head. Every time I walked by the knife drawer I tightened my fist. I would not reach for one. I would not. Knives didn't kill me as a child and they wouldn't now. Eventually I fell into a drunken stupor. I knew it was unattractive, my weaving back and forth to the fridge, tripping occasionally on the throw rugs, but at least I didn't die. I was keeping myself alive. That was my goal. I would live. And I did. I got through the night.

The next day I shuffled through breakfast, pushed the swollen door open with my shoulder and listened for any sounds coming from the shed. Nothing. The boys would be asleep for hours. I knew I should keep myself busy and wondered if I could leave them alone. Oh, for heaven's sake, I said to myself, they're twelve! I left cereal and bowls on the table and went to do the shopping. As I drove down the long empty road that ran along the spine of the peninsula, I felt as if a film of gray gauze had settled over my eyes. My heart was filled with despair. When I got to the corner store at the highway, I made a quick decision and pulled in at the phone booth. Maybe Richard would cheer me up. I dialed my husband at work, punching in numbers while swatting away mosquitoes.

"Can I please speak with Richard?" I waited while he came on the line. "Hi sweetie, how are you doing?

"Well, not as well as lucky you, doing nothing but reading on the beach."

Something inside me snapped. "Wait a minute. Just wait a minute. You think I'm having fun?" My voice was escalating.

"C'mon I..."

"C'mon what? I'm lucky? I'll tell you how lucky I am," I was screaming into the phone, "I'm so lucky that here comes a Mac truck, just when I feel like killing myself."

I threw down the receiver and ran toward the highway as the truck barrelled around the corner. The driver blew his horn and the bellow physically jolted me. I lost my footing and the dirt shoulder of the highway approached my face in slow motion as I fell forwards, hands outstretched. Next thing I knew I was sitting on the edge of the highway weeping and picking bits of gravel out of my knees and hands.

What had I done? Oh my god, what had I done? The kids. My husband. Richard. He'd be so worried.

I limped to the phone booth and called him back. "Sorry I said that. Sorry. I never would, you know." He wasn't to know how close I'd come. "I'll never do that again."

"I couldn't reach you. The phone booth doesn't receive calls. Your cell had no signal. I was so frightened. What have you been doing that has made you so upset, sweetie?"

"I don't know. Nothing." I was crying.

"What did you do last night?" Richard was infinitely patient.

"Nothing much. I read a bit." I wasn't going to tell him I got pissed to the gills.

"What did you read?"

"Blackwood's chart." The truth was out.

"Jesus, Sky! You are miles from nowhere. You have no supports. Your therapist is two thousand kilometres away. Don't read his god-damn chart."

He was shouting at me.

I hated shouting. It frightened me.

"Don't shout at me. Please don't shout. Is that what upset me?"

"Of course it is. Put it away. Listen to me. They're just words on paper. It's not real. It was then. It's not now. Don't read it. Put it away."

"Okay."

Richard quieted down, now that he knew I wouldn't read the chart. "How are the boys? Now that they're twelve they're pretty rambunctious. Can you manage?"

"Don't worry, honey. The kids are fine. Right now they're sleeping. I've set them up in the shed. They love it."

"You going to be home for your birthday? It is an important one, you know."

I was going to be fifty. Where had the time gone?

"Of course I will, honey." I'd make it to half a century if it killed me.

That afternoon, after I dropped the boys off at a neighbour's, I found my EMDR relaxation tape, lay on my bed, untangled the wires of my headphones from my Walkman, put them on and pressed play. I was soon asleep but was startled awake by a terrible nightmare. I paced around my living room, my hand grabbing at my throat. "I can't get air. Arm around neck. Can't breathe. Going to scream. Flip the flip. Flip the flip. Carving up my skin. He told me he loved me. He flipped me."

I sat down on the couch, hugging my body. Whispering to myself, "I'm not crazy. I'm sane. Very sane." I remembered Ann saying to me at one of our lunches, "You're not insane. What happened to you was insane. You are having a sane reaction to an insane event." I wasn't crazy. And despite the fact that I seemed much worse, I knew I was getting better. I was facing the truth. Some picnic.

After dinner the kids and I walked to the government wharf and watched the sunset. As usual, the boys chased each other around the end of the pier and, as usual, I shouted at them to stay away from the edge. The water at the end of the wharf gave me the creeps. It churned like a tornado and I quaked at the thought of anyone falling in, myself included.

As I approached the edge, my eyes were riveted to the dark swirling eddies of water. I forced myself to look up and watch the sun go down on the far shore. As it set, its rays pierced the filmy lens through which I looked and illuminated the darkened recesses of my brain with liquid gold. In that moment I felt the bright molten metal of the sun slide up and down my spine, like a forged sword. I felt so strong as I stood up perfectly straight. I wasn't going to fall into the water.

That night I grabbed just three beers and lined them up on the end table beside the couch. I wiggled my fingers at the rug, "Fooled ya. No trips to the fridge tonight."

At the top of a page I wrote "Swords and Water" and then scribbled away. Periodically my hands waved in the air as I pantomimed the end of the wharf and the setting sun. I was figuring out exactly what had happened to me as I watched the sunset. I didn't really know, but the line "you can't cut water with a sword and you can't break a sword with water" somehow meant a lot to me. Whatever. I would be fine.

CHAPTER 27

I SQUINTED MY EYES against the glare as I hiked out to the end of a local seaside national park, the Kejimkujik Adjunct. The water bottle in my fanny pack thumped against the small of my back as I hiked along the groomed trail. The sun was burning through the last wisps of late morning fog and I could feel its warmth through my sun hat. I marched quickly to the end of the point and made a wry face at my white socks and running shoes. Richard always laughed when I dressed like this. I was really looking forward to seeing him in a few days.

When I got to the ocean, I left the main trail and picked my way over a thin path through wild roses and sea grass toward the smooth surface of what everyone around called "Whaleback Rock." It seemed all the big rocks were called "Whaleback Rock."

I found my usual chair, a conveniently located throne of stone that faced the ocean. Before I sat down I emptied my fanny pack of my sandwich, somewhat squished, and the bottle of water. I settled onto the warm rock and looked at the silvery sea, mentally saying good-bye as I savoured my lunch. I was leaving Nova Scotia in the morning and had to brace myself for the College hearing in the early winter.

I had come here to the end of the point for a reason: I was going to burn beautiful images into my memory. They might come in handy. I blinked my eyes together, pretending I was a camera taking snapshots. I got good ones of the beach, rocks, sky, birds, and ocean. I knew I would steady myself on these mental photographs during the hearing while I told strangers intimate details about myself.

He'd *better* lose his license. All that exposure. So embarrassing.

As I worked a piece of food out of my teeth with my tongue, I fretted about my memory letting me down at crucial moments. I thought about how elusive memory was and noticed some black circles embedded in granite. Years ago I had overheard a geology professor from Dalhousie

University telling a group of environmentalists that these black circles were called "rock pipes" or brescia. The vertical pipes of hard rock had been formed when the lava-like center of the earth boiled up from deep miles below and bubbled into the roiling granite above. To me the black circles proved the power of the deep. They were time solidified and forever embedded in acknowledgement of the core of the earth. They were a testimony to the power of molten memory, the morphic resonance of long ago.

I listened to the seals sing while pondering the connection between rock pipes and memory. I crumpled my sandwich bag into a tiny little ball, tucked it into my fanny pack and wiped the crumbs off my hands. With a tentative finger I touched the rocky surface of a black circle. I shut my eyes in the dizzy recollection of touching David's soft soul and reminded myself I was now caressing the surface of Whaleback Rock, not Blackwood's heart.

I forced myself to feel the rock and be in the here and now at the end of the Keji Adjunct, not in his office. As I ran my hand over the surface of the rock with my eyes closed I couldn't distinguish the rock pipes from the granite. I found this somehow reassuring. I slowly turned my head back and forth as I caressed the rock and listened to the seals sing. Their haunting voices rose and fell on the curling mist and I thought they sounded like ghosts.

I knew then, in that singular moment that was caught between the rock and the seals, there was no way I'd ever forget what Blackwood had done to me. My memory was not going to fail me when I was questioned on the stand. I could dissociate to another planet, my Post Traumatic Stress Disorder could blow me right away, but the memories would boil up from my depths and wail like ghosts.

I felt the rock dig into the palms of my hands as I pushed against it to stand up. I hastily looked around. Had anybody seen me? I knew I looked demented, blinking my eyes taking pretend photographs and rubbing my hands over the surface of Whaleback Rock while tilting my head back and forth with my eyes shut. I shook my head and laughed at myself. I couldn't wait to see Richard.

The next morning the boys and I headed out early, lunches and dinners packed into cooler bags for the journey back to Toronto. The two-day drive on the long black ribbon of highway through the bush was punctuated by pee stops, snacks, and green exit signs with tantalizing names.

I thought of Ann and what she had told me over many lunches about the College's hearings. Once a week Ann would give her various warnings, her mouth full of western sandwiches washed down with numerous coffees laced with scotch. Through a veil of cigarette smoke she would caution me, "You know you're going to be turned into a nut/slut whacko. That's what they do. There is no defence for what he did, so they attack the victim. You will be the one on trial, not him. Remember that."

I gripped the wheel, bracing myself against being attacked at the hearing. Ann had told me this would happen. And I believed her. Ann had laughed, "Just watch, Blackwood's lawyers are going to trot out old Dr. Merriweather as their expert witness. He'll tell everyone you're so evil, you boil baby rabbits for breakfast, like in that movie, *Fatal Attraction*. That you have a Borderline Personality Disorder. That's what he did to me when I reported the psychiatrist."

And I, in my innocence, had asked, "What's a Borderline Personality Disorder?"

"Thought you'd never ask. Probably the worst diagnosis a person can get. Untreatable. Life long. Incurable. A sentence of madness."

"Oh," I'd said.

Good thing Blackwood wrote everything down in his chart. No arguing with that!

I also knew that unfortunately all victims of repeated, long-term sexual abuse do go crazy, in some way. I sure did. It's how I coped. Talking aloud in my car kept me alive. It kept me from thinking about what happened. I was busy. A pretty healthy reaction to a very sick situation, if you asked me. Crazy? They would have a field day with me. Three years of playing The Blue Car Game? Circling Blackwood's house? Stealing his garbage? Yeah, but I lived.

When I got to Montreal I drove down into the tunnel under the St. Lawrence and steeled myself against the neon lighting as it rhythmically pulsed through my windshield. Ann's words rang in my ears. "He gets three lawyers. You don't get one. You are just a witness for the College. Nothing more. You don't count. Remember that. The lawyer you're talking to is not your lawyer. She doesn't care about you. She is the lawyer for the College. She cares only about the College. Don't forget that. You are all alone." Ann had pointed her chipped nail at me. With each pulsing light in the tunnel I kept hearing, "You are all alone, you are all alone, you are all alone."

I knew the defence would have access to every scrap of paper about the case at the College, and the College would be in the dark. Judith, the College investigator, had told me that. She had said, "They get everything, we get nothing."

This would mean that the defence's ability to build a case would be facilitated and the College wouldn't have the same advantage. The College wouldn't have any surprise opportunities to prove Blackwood was a liar. What a biased system.

I was adding it all up in my head as I drove. In my mind I had two columns, one for the defence and the other for the College. The defence column was full of advantages and the College's side had nothing. Hmm, I thought, seems like we have a little systemic prejudice here. I barked a laugh right out loud. The boys' heads shot up at the sound, then just as quickly went back to their video game.

The exits for Kingston finally came and went and jumbled thoughts tossed around in my mind. That man had ruined ten years of my life. The odds of winning at the College were infinitesimal. But then again, only one in over two thousand complaints actually make it to a hearing, and mine had. So maybe I would win. Maybe, maybe. But my character would be assassinated. Could I take it? I knew my nerves were shot. Fried. I was a basket case, not a prosecution case. Old joke.

Ha, I barked. The boys didn't even look up.

"The lawyers representing Blackwood at the College hearing get my psychiatric chart," I told Barbara, dismayed by the news.

"I know. I've been to meetings."

Barbara had been to meetings? For me? I took that in slowly as Barbara's face floated in and out of view. Why was I dissociating? Shit, I thought, it was because Barbara was supporting me. Why was this so frightening?

"So, you'll give my chart to them?"

"I argued it was not in your best interest to have your chart exposed."

"I thought if I were suicidal a judge wouldn't allow it. Why are they getting it?"

"I don't know, I told them you were suicidal. Ask your lawyer."

"Where were the meetings? Here in your office?"

"No, downtown."

I was flabbergasted that Barbara would do this. No one in my whole life had protected me from anything. "Why did you go? Why are you protecting me? You know I'm an ugly piece of shit."

"It seemed like the right thing to do."

"Oh." I could hardly breathe.

That night I sat in my office, a pad of paper in front of me, and a beer at my side. I remembered how I had suddenly become frightened and dissociated in Barbara's office because she had stepped up to bat for me. I began my usual whispering. "I feel like, I don't know, I feel like I've been crawling out of a black hole in outer space ever since I met Barbara. Finally I've reached the edge of the hole. So I sit here perched." I rocked back and forth. "Wavering back and forth, to dive or not to dive into the universe towards another human being.

"Now I feel myself dancing back from the edge of the hole where a camera is filming in slow motion, the image jittery and in reverse. I'm watching the film." My hands became a running movie projector. "And I see where I was and where I wasn't when I sat in Barbara's office." I stopped running the projector and shook my finger. "I know what I have to do. I have to push myself away from the edge of the black hole."

I wrote all this down furiously and then looked up. "I'm free-falling, flipping over and screaming towards earth. My fingernails are scratching the edge of the sky. I can see my body burst into flames from the friction of the fall. It's some sort of cleansing ritual. I'm falling so fast I'm shattering the sound barrier."

I rubbed my forehead. "Now I have to land. How? I have to bend the air so I can direct my burning body to land my bones on the softest place around."

I wrote this down, read it, tapped the page and then said, "And that would be Barbara. I will land on Barbara. This is about trust. I will trust my psychiatrist. Ah ha!"

I was so angry about the defence getting my current psychiatric chart that I called my lawyer for the civil case. "Why did the defence get

Barbara's chart? Barbara argued I was suicidal and it wasn't in my best interest for my chart to be exposed. It would threaten me. I have been suicidal."

"Yes, but it was only three times."

Jesus.

I called Ann. "I asked my civil case lawyer why the defence got my chart and she said it was because I was suicidal only three times."

Ann laughed, her squawk deafening in my ear, "Write a book called *Stupid Things Lawyers Say*."

CHAPTER 28

FOR THE NEXT THREE weeks Judith and I sat in various board-rooms around the College building, day after day, preparing for the hearing by going over every single entry that Blackwood had made in his chart on me. We filtered through all the pages of evidence. My calendars. Receipts for gifts. Phone bills. And the seven hundred and eighty poems. In the pile of letters was the one I had sent to Cindy. "Wasn't from me!" I lied. The print outs of emails included the one I had sent her about Blackwood's affairs. "That guy sure gets around," I quipped.

My nights were filled with nightmares of a lion stalking me and nuzzling his mane against my soft belly while I lay down in a cave, waiting for him to eat me. My days were filled with large bodies of water, through which I tried to navigate, my body weighted and somehow separated from the world of people who lived in air. Every now and then the water would suddenly disappear and my world would spin so fast that the friction of my inner life would rub against reality, turning my existence into steaming smoke.

But I knew I looked normal in my jeans and running shoes, sitting at the boardroom table, munching on delicious sandwiches provided by the College. If Judith asked, I always said I was okay.

I also knew that Judith knew I wasn't. But Judith would pretend that I was. This was how she preserved what few shreds of dignity I could keep from sliding through my fingers. Every now and then she would stop typing and speak about more normal things, and we would laugh while she rolled her eyes about this and that.

"He isn't a normal person, you know Judith."

"Clearly," she said sarcastically.

"I mean, there's something about him that's just kind of, I don't know, I can't put my finger on it."

"Well, I can." Judith leaned forward and looked at me around the stack of papers in front of her. She lowered her voice, her telltale sign that she was going to give me some information that I shouldn't really have. "I will never forget being in his office. Of all the doctors I have served notice on, I will never forget him. He is like an evil force." Judith wrapped her arms around herself, as if to protect her body from his awful energy. "I get goose bumps when I think of him. His eyes? They are something else. Like a wild animal or something."

"A lion."

Finally Judith and I had finished going through Blackwood's chart, the evidence, and the poems. We stood outside on the corner chatting and laughing in the clear fall air. We had done a good job, raking through the memories of what had happened in that office, day by day, chart entry by chart entry. As we were saying good-bye Judith held out her hand for me to shake.

"Well, good job Kathy, see you soon."

I shook Judith's hand, "Thanks. It's been fun preparing for the hearing." Oh my god, I could feel her hand!

By the time I got back to my car in the parking lot, I was looking at my hand and weeping. I sat behind my steering wheel, tears streaming down my face. "I have been touched. I could feel it. I could feel it in my heart." I placed my right arm over my heart. "Judith touched my heart. For the first time in over ten years I can feel touch. I am back in my body. What a gift!" I sobbed. "She touched me. I've been touched."

I cried for a few minutes while I kept touching my hand and looking at it in front of my face. It was connected to me. Finally I took a deep breath and looked around to see if anyone was watching me talk to my hand in my car.

I pointed to my ear and made small circles. Cuckoo.

That night I sat in my office and wrote at the top of a page, "The Touch of a Handshake." I took a sip of my beer and started whispering, "Blackwood's fingerprints stayed in the memory of my cells." I clasped my hands together. "I can feel the pain in the soft flesh on my fingers. I can feel the pain slowly bubble through the thick wet memory of how I touched him and how he touched me. I forbade myself to feel touch because he had betrayed me so deeply. My hands hurt for years."

I took a sip of beer.

And then I replayed shaking Judith's hand goodbye. "I let myself feel who she was. I could feel her integrity and human kindness. It all hummed up my arm to my heart." With my left hand I followed the path of the feeling up my arm to my heart.

And then I relived how the pain had gone away and I could feel my fingers. I entwined them softly. "I can feel my fingers. The pain is gone. It's gone! All because of a touch in a handshake."

I put my pen on the paper and hurriedly wrote it down. When I was finished I looked at my poem and whispered, "I vow, one day, to send this poem to Judith. How can I ever thank her?"

The hearing was scheduled for a few weeks away and the lawyer for the College, Berka Winters, started to prepare me for the questions she would ask me while I was on the stand. We had a series of meetings with Judith, Berka, and me.

Berka asked me question after question and I answered them with my hands on the table in front of me to steady myself in the face of the awful answers and my overwhelming guilt. I knew that the practice, although gruelling, was a good thing to do. Because of my Post Traumatic Stress Disorder I would lose my focus if I became frightened, but the repetition of telling the event seemed to be taming the ordeal to a manageable level of fear.

But Berka's last question about me masturbating on the floor slid into me like a knife. She asked, "Whose idea was that?"

I could feel my shame suffocating all the dignity I had left. I broke down and whispered, "Mine." A sob escaped my throat. "That's the problem. It was all my fault."

I wanted to die as I spoke what I thought was the truth. My overwhelming shame had completely erased my memory of Blackwood's words, "You do that."

Nobody said anything while I hung my head and stared at the gray Formica table top. My guilt tumbled into the silence and careened around the room. I knew the case would be lost because it was all my fault.

When I looked up I saw that the blood had been pressed out of Berka's hands as she pushed them down on the table. She was staring at me, her mouth a blue-gray slit across her face. The vein in her forehead

. thought she was furious at me. She would lose the case
as so evil.

jaw barely moved as she spoke, "If there is one thing I am
to say to you, it is this." She paused, took a deep breath, and
I aced myself against the force of her wrath. I was going to get a
lecture like I'd never had before.

"*This was not your fault.*"

I looked at her and shook my head. Berka didn't understand. But
then she repeated what she had said, her voice raised. "*This was not
your fault.*" Her words jumped around the square white room like
random squash balls pinging off the walls. "He was the doctor. You
were the patient. This was his fault." Berka repeated it again, her words
bouncing into my wall of guilt. "This was *his* fault!" Her anger wasn't
at me at all, it was at the doctor!

I didn't quite believe her, but in that moment I knew I could pretend
to. I could act as if Berka were right. I even toyed with the idea that she
might be. And because Berka was "One-To-Be-Obeyed," I nodded.

Berka spent a full week with me going over the questions she was
going to ask at the hearing. Every night I would go home, a shroud of
guilt enveloping my mind.

Drinking helped.

"I can't lie under oath. I just can't. I feel so guilty, my soul feels black.
I don't know what to do." I was confessing to Marion.

"What are you guilty about? That, 'it's all my fault' crap?'"

"No, I lied. It was such a tiny lie. Well, two lies. But I don't know
what to do."

"If you stick to the truth then the story will be told. What did you
lie about?"

"I can't tell you. They were such little lies. I mean, it's of no relevance,
but I just don't think I can lie. It would be impossible to catch me in
them. But I feel so terrible. "

"Sleep on it. You'll know what to do in the morning."

The next morning I knew what I had to do. I had to tell the truth.

I went to my scheduled meeting with Judith and Berka, a cloak of
seriousness tightly pulled around me.

"I have something to tell you. I can't lie. I have lied to you both."
I took a deep breath. "I was the one who sent the warning email to

Cindy. I also wrote her that letter."

A dark shadow lifted from the corner of my mind.

"You sure had me fooled," said Judith sympathetically. "Victims lie. They always do. They have to. They think it makes them look better, but it makes them look worse. People shouldn't be embarrassed about their behaviour. They act the way they do because of what the doctor did to them. It's not their fault. Why did you send the email?"

"I needed Cindy to know that David wasn't to be trusted. I somehow needed to protect her from what had happened to me. I knew I was going to report him and I wanted her safely out of the way, I didn't want her to be hurt."

Berka, on the other hand, didn't like being lied to, not two weeks before the hearing. Again the vein in the middle of her forehead throbbed and I knew trouble was afoot. "If I decide at the end of the day that your testimony is unreliable, I will counsel the panel to disregard it. I have been trying to decide whether or not to put you on the stand."

I was aghast. I mentally repeated her sentences to myself three times so I would never forget them. What did she mean, *unreliable*? I was too bonkers to testify? *Fuck her.* I had proof! Every word I had said in my statement to the College, every allegation, had been corroborated by Blackwood's chart, proving that my memory was impeccable, that I wasn't nuts. But what Berka had just said made me understand that there was deep-rooted prejudice and misunderstanding about the impact of sexual abuse in the legal system.

I was furious. But I could fight back. At moments like this I was kept sane by knowing I could write a book about the fucking goddamn prejudice. I pressed my lips shut.

And then I inwardly grimaced. I'd also have to tell the readers of my book to never, ever, *ever* lie. Big mistake.

CHAPTER 29

I WAS SCOOTING UP the expressway to Yorkdale Mall, remembering the times I couldn't drive on the highway. But look at me now! Here I was, driving like no tomorrow, off to deal with my clothing issues before the hearing. I was so much better! How long had it been since I bought clothes? More to the point, how long had it been since I handed in that Letter of Complaint? Almost a year. Wow! And the *Registered Health Professions Act* said a hearing had to happen within one hundred and fifty days. Yeah, right. If the College couldn't pay attention to that pretty basic requirement, it didn't bode well for how they'd behave during a hearing. I shook off the ominous thoughts gathering in my mind like storm clouds as I pulled into a parking space and focused on what I needed to do before the hearing.

First of all, I needed to shop! I stood in front of a rack of skirts. What on earth was in fashion? Above the knee? Below the knee? How on earth would I know? Fashion had been the last thing on my mind. I gave up and bought pants. As I walked through the mall giddily victorious with my purchases, an undercurrent of reality tugged at my euphoria. It was all so ridiculous. I almost died and here I am, pleased as punch with cheap suits. No, I corrected myself, "law suits."

Ha ha.

When I got home, I fired off two emails. Ann had told me to remind the press about the hearing. One went to Dan Pascussi, the reporter who had written the story about Blackwood not complying with his Order of Restrictions. The other went to Natty Hitchens, a columnist for a national paper. A friend had told me that Natty was a champion of women's rights. That could be helpful.

My emails said that not many women reported doctor abuse and I hoped that if they read about it maybe more would come forward. I said doctor abuse was a huge problem and needed to be stopped. I warned the reporters that I would be turned into a nut/slut whacko, and thank heavens, Dr. Blackwood had written it all down!

Then I got a support group together. I knew that I would be dissociating, depersonalizing, de-everything, and it would really help to anchor myself if familiar faces were in the crowd. I didn't want Richard to go. It wasn't that I was worried he would punch Blackwood out in some sort of macho rage, Richard wasn't like that, but I just didn't want him to hear how I'd been harmed. It would really upset him. So, I called fifteen of my friends to support me during the hearing. I asked each of them for either a morning stint, a lunch break, or an afternoon session. I was so lucky; no one said no.

On the morning of the hearing I stood in front of my mirror and critically eyed myself in my new black pant suit with the pale orange blouse. I felt like hallowe'en candy.

"You look nice." Marion was driving me down for the first day of the hearing.

"I clean up good." We didn't say another word all the way downtown.

I peered through the open door and saw the hearing room was filling up. To my right I could see the press: all four Toronto papers were represented, the journalists gossiping while they waited for their story. I could see the cherry wood desk where I would sit, with its snake-necked microphone and glass of water. My palms began to sweat. Deep in the room was Judith, her piles of evidence stacked beside her.

Pain flashed through me like a sharp current of electricity: paper didn't really matter. It was just paper: calendars, bills, receipts, letters, poems. None of it mattered. That wasn't the evidence. The true evidence was my body.

My skin had been covered with his fingerprints. I wanted to stand naked in front of the judging panel and shout, "Look, here, and here, look at this, there isn't an inch of skin on my body he didn't touch." But unfortunately, this evidence had become so hot it had burnt up and disappeared into smoke. I had become nothing. Perhaps I should tell the panel that the prosecution had nothing as their evidence.

Giddiness welled up in me. Was I becoming hysterical?

And straight ahead was David's back. I recognized his yellowish skin shining through the bald spot on the crown of his head. Familiar tufts of unruly hair sprouted from his neck and made me want to shout, "get a haircut, will ya!" Flecks of dandruff dusted his shoulders and I swallowed the disgust that rose like bile in my throat.

As I stared at his back something seemed off kilter. What was it? Something was very different. What on earth was it? What was wrong with this picture? Suddenly, blindingly, the answer came to me like an epiphany: he was *short!*

I whispered to the Victim Support Person, Hanna Turner, "I can't believe how small he is. How short." I caught Marion's eye across the room and cocked my head towards Blackwood while putting my thumb and forefinger together as if measuring an inch. I mouthed the word "short." Marion thought I meant his penis and burst out laughing.

Hanna said, "Almost all victims say that. The doctor becomes diminished somehow through the process."

"Be that as it may, my heart is just racing," I said to Hanna.

"You'll be fine. He looks awful. His suit doesn't even fit. Look at the puckering around his shoulders," said Hanna.

"He dresses really badly," I whispered, remembering that stupid white thread dangling from the crotch of his blue pants.

"It's probably his goal to look pathetic," said Hanna.

Fear prickled the back of my neck. "That's the game he's going to play? He is going to be *my* victim?"

Ann had warned me about this, but I hadn't believed it. She'd said, "They'll have no defence you know, Sky," Ann's mouth had been full of a western sandwich. "So they'll turn him into *your* victim, just watch."

I felt my skin contract as I walked behind him in his rumpled blue suit, the sleeves too short.

His hands!

Suddenly I could feel them touching me everywhere, carving his name on my flesh. My stomach lurched. Was I going to throw up?

He's a lion, I thought. He's going to eat me. I'm going to have nightmares. I know it. I remembered his oral sex psycho-dramas and could see the pattern in the awful tapestry moving in the shadows behind him like black flames. I remembered crying and him bundling me into his arms, assuring me it was good therapy. Yeah, right, that's why we were here today.

I sat at my allocated desk, head down. I simply could not look at him. Judith knew it was difficult for me to see Blackwood and positioned herself so she was blocking him from my view. If he shifted in his chair, Judith would readjust her position to keep him out of my sight. I was quite certain it hurt her back to be sitting the way she was and was grateful to her for helping me.

The room suddenly went quiet and the proceedings began. Berka started asking me routine background questions. University? Children? Marriage? Career? I tried to keep my voice from wavering. Then the questions became more difficult and I felt like they were being pitched at me, one after another. "Could you please describe to the panel some of Dr. Blackwood's psycho-dramas," asked Berka.

I watched myself as if I were in a horror movie while I choked out the words that he had an erection while he stood behind my back, touching my erogenous zones to rewire me. I showed the panel how he had placed one hand around my neck and the other over my mouth so I wouldn't scream while he acted out anally raping me. I mumbled how he had watched me masturbating on the dirty floor of his office while I told him sexual fantasies. I went off into space while my mouth opened and shut, telling stories I didn't want to know. My mind made sure I wasn't there.

Finally there was a break. Everyone stood up while the panel exited the room. I looked over them carefully, trying to size them up. The first person who passed me was a woman who had come from Ottawa to open the hearing. The look she gave me was one of compassion and understanding, her soft blue eyes seemingly melting into mine.

Next came a stocky, military kind of guy with a pock-marked face and a short buzzcut. He gave me the willies. I knew his type, a self-righteous do-gooder who pretended to be respectful of women but really enjoyed controlling them. I could smell cruelty in the air around him as he walked by.

Then there was the Chair of the panel, a compact and agile heart surgeon who probably had been berated all his life for being moral and studious. I knew he would do the right thing, I could tell he was smart. He would understand. His face was beet red. He was probably incensed that while he operated on people in life and death circumstances here was this runt of a doctor who billed OHIP for hugging.

Then came a short woman who moved like a warship. Although she didn't glance at me, I could sense as she brushed past that she was a feminist and that Blackwood disgusted her. I wished I had this woman's self-confidence, so evident as she plowed through the air, the bosom of her bow cutting through bullshit.

The fifth member of the five-person panel was a short, corpulent man. I knew he would never allow Blackwood to lose his license. He looked just plain mean and dismissive of women. As he waddled past me I sensed arrogance and judgment. I tallied it up, three against two.

I could win.

Once the panel had filed out of the room, everyone else was allowed to leave. I walked slowly towards the door and passed Natty Hitchens, the columnist from the national paper, who was still jotting down notes. I smiled at her. "Thank you for coming."

Natty glanced up and smirked, "I wouldn't have missed it for the world!"

Her voice slid across my nerves like fingernails on a chalkboard. I looked at the woman and felt a shiver flash through my heart. I thought anxiously, what have I done? She had that arrogant sneer, that derogatory bearing of a woman hater. Was she prejudiced against victims of assault? How *could* I have asked her to the hearing? It would be my downfall. I just knew Natty's reporting would be biased in favour of Blackwood. I saw Natty look at my shoes and make a cryptic note on her pad. The decimation had begun, from the feet up.

As I walked through the hearing room doors, Hanna Turner leapt up and circled around me like a mother hen, leading the way towards our reserved waiting room, protecting me from an encounter with Blackwood. "You know, most victims don't have a single friend. It is very unusual that you have so many friends in the audience."

"I'm so grateful they could come." My heart melted as I remembered how I had lost my train of thought during one of the questions and in a panic looked up, only to see Fay, who had replaced Marion for the afternoon shift. Fay had been there at the very beginning, encouraging me at lunch that day when I handed in my Letter of Complaint. Now she was gesturing instructions to me, her chest exaggeratedly going in and out, reminding me to breathe.

After the break I did my best answering Berka's pointed questions, but I could feel myself fading into a foggy nightmare. By the time I got home that night fear was slicing at the inside of my skin. I was so tired of my skin hurting.

I could hear Richard's car pull up to the curb in front of our house and I flung myself into his arms the minute he walked in the door. "I'm so glad you're home."

"How did it go, sweetie?"

"Oh my god, it was awful. Blackwood really gives me the creeps."

Richard hung up his coat and stuck his finger into a strawberry sauce I had made to go over ice cream. "Was the press there?"

"Oh yeah, were they ever. That Hitchens, watch out. I can feel it."

He licked his finger. "But I thought she was pro-women's rights."

"Me too, but I just got off the phone with Ella and guess what? Hitchens was her best friend in high school and I think she hates me because now I'm Ella's friend."

He wrapped his arms around me. "You're almost done Sky, and good for you."

Halfway through my week on the stand, I had to see Barbara. I was in trouble. "I feel as if I am walking across a frozen lake that is cracking and booming under me. It's as if I can feel the ice shift, like tectonic plates, into a sudden clarity."

"Yes," said Barbara, writing.

"My mind is scuttling across the ice as the mane of the lion brushes my belly."

"You're frightened."

"I am such a bad person," I paused, "and it's my fault. It's my fault and I am going to fall through the ice and the lion is going to eat me."

Then I sat back in my chair and shuddered. Barbara looked up.

I don't know why, but for the second time in my many years of seeing her, I asked, "Do you care about me?"

Barbara gave an almost disbelieving shake of her shoulders and said, "Of course I do."

"Oh, okay. Just checking. I won't fall through. Right, Barbara? Right?"

"You're not bad, Kathy."

A few days later Berka's questions for the prosecution were finally done. I drove around to various newspaper boxes, grabbing copies of all the different papers. I read with disbelief as I thumbed through the crackling pages. My skin burned with shame as the minute details about what had happened in that office were gleefully, sadistically, revealed.

I called Richard at work. "I can't believe what they're writing. I am so upset."

"Just don't let the children see the papers, Kathy."

"You're not kidding."

Natty Hitchens was the worst. Her malice towards me knew no bounds. She violated the publication ban on the hearing! How could she? The ban stated, 'no person shall publish ...any information that could disclose the identity of the complainant...'" But because of Hitchens, the whole world knew that Blackwood's victim was 50 years old, had a small frame and red hair, was a writer, and lived in Toronto. They knew I had three children, was university educated, had a summer cottage, and a pond in my Toronto backyard. Just to make sure I was identified, Hitchens wrote the final detail that would cinch the deal: Richard's birth date. It had come out during the testimony. She'd reported that I'd said that Blackwood had taught me foreplay on Richard's birthday, July 4th. No one but me could fit all her identifying details and be married to a guy with that exact birth date. Of course I would be identified. And I was.

My phone rang off the hook.

CHAPTER 30

I T WAS NOW THE defence's turn to cross-examine me. Within minutes of being on the stand I started to shake deep in my core. Robert Keating, Blackwood's lawyer, stood hunched in a perpetual question mark in front of me. His questions were making me dissociate. I was watching myself as if I were in an old grainy movie as I went over the past. His thin face was folded into his bony shoulders, and he looked like a shark, waiting to strike. Behind him sat the hapless Blackwood, lurking in the dark shadows of the room. I watched Keating dart back and forth, lunging forward when he asked a question, and then reeling me back with his net ready.

I had been instructed by Berka to wait for the question, to speak only in response to a question, and to answer the question briefly and succinctly. I was not to volunteer any additional information. Nothing. This seemed simple enough. But by the time Keating got around to Ann and her expedition to Blackwood's office, I couldn't even understand the question, no less answer it.

"So, you and Ann Foster took it upon yourselves to police Dr. Blackwood."

Was that a question? If it were, what did it mean? Police? "Police" is a noun. How did I police Blackwood? Was this a ritual that I had forgotten about? One involving uniforms?

"I don't understand the question, could you please reword it?"

"Did you and Ann take it upon yourselves to police Dr. Blackwood?"

Why was he talking about Ann? Ann had gone to Blackwood as a patient. He was required by law to keep his patients' names confidential. Why did he keep breaking laws? And there was that word again, that "police."

"I'm sorry, I don't understand the question, could you please repeat it?"

Keating just looked at me, exasperated, and moved on to the next question. While he was asking it, I suddenly understood the previous question. Keating wanted to know if Ann and I had taken it upon ourselves to *monitor* Blackwood. At this point I wanted to shout, "Well, somebody had to, idiot," but by then, of course, it was too late, and I had to ask for the next question to be repeated.

I wasn't doing very well.

Keating was relentless in his questions and I had difficulty keeping up. My mind was trembling in a far corner of my skull, barely functioning. I tried to focus on my friends in the chairs in front of me and every time I looked up I saw I was loved and supported. I could feel it.

I could also feel cold sweat dripping into the satiny lining of my new suit. Just shit, I thought.

But now there were only four members on the panel. Shouldn't that be illegal? Didn't the *Regulated Health Professionals Act* say there had to be an odd number to avoid a tie? I would look it up. The kind doctor from Ottawa had bowed out because she was very ill. I knew that both the military guy and the corpulent fellow would side with Blackwood. They would be fooled into thinking he was not a predator and had merely gotten in over his head because he only wanted to help me. They would believe I was a difficult patient and he, poor man, had suffered from counter-transference in his desire to help me. Without five people on the panel tipping the balance in my favour, I knew that Blackwood would not lose his license.

I wanted Berka to call me to the stand again for the prosecution. She had done nothing to present me in a favourable light. Not once had she asked, "You were so upset by what happened, what did you do next?" She had not brought out the truth: that Blackwood enjoyed humiliating me and that his abuse of power over me was his aphrodisiac while he toyed with my body. Nor did she bring out the truth that Blackwood erotically teased me daily and then rejected my erotic response to humiliate me. That he "gently" stated his "boundaries" while pressing his erection against me. All this, so I would beg for sex. She did not bring out the truth that Blackwood had sexually tortured me. That he had driven me crazy.

I sent Berka an email, imploring her to expose the truth and put me back on the stand. Berka's response? I was chastised for writing such an email! She wrote, "I want to remind you that when you email me, or call me, if you provide me with any new information about the case, I am obliged to disclose it to the defence."

I stared at the email as the letters vibrated, every so slightly, on my computer screen.

Whose side was Berka on?

The defence's cross-examination continued. A bank of windows shone with the whiteness of a wintry sun behind the four people on the panel, showing only their body shapes in dark silhouette. While I was being questioned I tried to feel the warmth of the sun, hoping it would stop my insides from trembling.

I was being questioned about masturbating on Blackwood's office floor.

Keating asked me, "Whose idea was that?"

"Mine. It was my idea." I shivered and told a roomful of people that I had asked to be sexually abused. It was all my fault. Everything bad that had happened to me all my life had been my fault. This was my truth, and I had to tell the truth. My inner truth submerged the facts: I had utterly suppressed Blackwood's "Would an orgasm help you?" and his "you do that" as well as his "I'm glad you know what's good for you," his "fantasy gets you ready for the real thing." I had buried our negotiated contracts deep in my mind.

Keating rubbed his hands together with glee and curled his lips in what he probably thought was a smile.

In front of me were my three therapists' charts, bound and photocopied, waiting like steel traps. I looked at them warily. What on earth had I said that warranted their very white and shining appearance here? How was Keating going to turn my words to my therapists into as-sassination bullets?

Ann had warned me that the College would not defend me. I looked at the charts. What? They'd be used to *turn* me into a crazy person? I already *was* a crazy person.

Keating picked up a chart and pointed with a scaly finger to an entry where he said I had asked Barbara never to write in my chart that I had a Borderline Personality Disorder. I was floored and answered that Barbara had told me she would never write any diagnosis in her chart because she didn't like to use labels, that he had read the entry incorrectly.

Berka jumped up and began a very long legal argument about the relevance of third party records because they were too wide open to interpretation. I was ushered out of the room while Berka struggled against Keating over whether or not I could be dragged through my therapy charts. I sat for two hours in one of the College's boardrooms and waited anxiously for the arguments to be over.

Suddenly there was a knock on the door. I was summoned back in.

Berka had won the argument! Hundreds of pages in the charts were out! Good for her! Had a precedent been set? Would medical charts be out for future victims? The College *had* protected me, if only a little, but they had. Ann had been wrong.

Keating was left referring to just one skimpy piece of paper: the test Maggie had given me to determine the extent of my dissociative disorder. Apparently this was kosher because it didn't rely upon third party interpretation. He waved it in the air like a victory flag and drew attention to the slashes on the lines.

"Did you make these marks?"

"Yes." I remembered with shame how I couldn't figure out the instructions to the test, how I had to read them over and over before they made sense.

Keating placed the piece of paper in front of me and zeroed in on the questions that had to do with memory.

"How often did you indicate that you couldn't remember how you had arrived somewhere?"

This didn't look good. Here was the proof, offered in my own hand, the little slashes like score marks for the defence. The print vibrated and I squinted my eyes so I could read through the now familiar yellow haze. "Ninety percent of the time."

Keating gloated. He had destroyed my credibility.

Berka jumped up and waved another piece of paper in the air. This was a second test Maggie had administered to me after a month of EMDR therapy. Berka thrust the paper under my nose. "Are these your answers?"

"Yes." The tremors inside me were getting worse. Did it show?

"I would like the panel to note that the slashes on the memory question lines indicate her memory was almost one hundred percent."

What was all this quibbling about? My memory was irrelevant. He'd written everything down.

And then Keating stood up, tapped his papers together and announced his questions were over. What? Only two hours of questions? But then again, Berka's lack of questions about the truth had already effectively destroyed me. My whole body was shaking as if I were living through a massive earthquake. I could barely get out of the witness seat and staggered out through what looked like, to me, a crooked door frame.

I crumpled into a chair in the waiting room. I slowly lifted my hand to my cheek and touched the puffy shadows under my eyes. I looked at my fingers. They were wet. The realization that I was crying percolated through my vibrating terror into my consciousness. Shouldn't I hear myself sobbing? Shouldn't I feel my shoulders shaking? But no, the tears just kept falling out of my eyes and rolling down my face. I didn't know where they came from. How did one cry yet not feel?

I muttered to myself to get a grip. Okay, how was I? First of all, was I alive? Yes, I could hear my heart. Good sign. But I couldn't see. Were my eyes shut? Must be. In the blackness I could feel my forehead pressing against my fingers. I must have my head in my hand. I could feel a terrible shaking. What was it? An earthquake? God, I was cold! Someone gave me a coat. It was my coat. I stroked it softly and draped it right over my head. I sat underneath the tent of my coat and could smell the soft perfume of my shampoo. I didn't care what anyone thought.

I sat in the small witness room at the College of Physicians and Surgeons of Ontario with my brown coat over my head. It was so dark. It felt like there was a volcano inside me. That's what was shaking. A swirling combustion of memory exploded. The cave was blowing up. I was lying on the skin of the earth and could feel a volcano erupting. A very bad thing was going to happen. No, a very bad thing was happening. The lion was screaming. I pulled the coat tighter over my head. I didn't want to watch what was flickering on the projector screen of my eyelids.

It was so hard to breathe. I was trapped under the ice. How did I get there? Then I knew. The volcano blew me off the earth and under the ice. Right. Happens all the time. Made sense to me. God, was I crazy? No, I *knew* I wasn't underwater. I couldn't breathe simply because a coat was over my head. What must the women in the room think? I didn't care.

I had to look at what I saw. I cringed; an image was dancing. Grotesquely contorting in pain. It was a lion, all bloody. Black flickering shadows were leaping behind my eyes. There was a deep red ghost of a lion dancing on my eyelids. I watched in horrid fascination. The red ghost lion was dancing in dark blood flames. Maybe the water under the ice would put the fire out. Maybe he'd burn up.

Stop it, I thought to myself. Stop it. Was I nuts? No. What happened to me was nuts. I said it again and again to myself like a mantra. *What happened to me was nuts, I'm not nuts. What happened to me was nuts, I'm not nuts.*

I thought I was going to throw up.

I didn't. I never did.

What was that noise? I could hear breathing. Was it me breathing? No, I was drowning under the ice. Definitely not breathing. It was the women. I could hear the women in the room with me. I wasn't alone. They were waiting for me. But I wasn't going to take the coat off my head. Not yet.

I could feel myself floating up towards them from under the ice. I had to, I could feel their love float from their souls, wrap around me, and lift me up and up from under the ice. As I got nearer the surface the water became clearer. I couldn't see the lion anymore. I was rising toward the surface of the sea. The ice had melted away. It was light. I could hear their love breathing in and out like surf echoing on a beach. I could feel the waves caress me as I surfaced.

I was jolted out of my underwater nightmare by a sudden revelation. I whispered into the polyester lining of my winter coat, "Holy shit."

Oops. I hoped the women didn't hear.

I could *feel* being loved. Without being touched. I sat very still. It was true. Through the soft feathers of my down winter coat I could feel being loved by the women sitting with me in the witness room. I hugged the coat tighter to me while I basked in their gentleness.

It was time to take the coat off my head. I decided to act as if nothing had happened at all. I lifted it off, put it neatly on my lap and patted down my flyaway hair. I was composed.

"There."

In unison the two women said, "There."

I was done with being under the ice. I was done with the lion. The women had been waiting for me above the ice. One was Hanna. The other was my daughter's art teacher, Ruth. These women did not know me well, but they loved me anyway. They were so kind. I was loved. I could actually feel it. It was over.

I asked Hanna, "Did I say on the stand about Blackwood looking like a lion and pretending to eat me? In the dark? His office was like a cave. Did I say that? A black cave?"

"You did. You did a good job. You said it. You told the truth."

"Good. It's over." I sighed, my breath trembling on my lips. "This is the last time he'll make me cry."

"You did a good job."

"Thank you for loving me, Hanna, Ruth."

"You're welcome," they both said together.

And just like that I re-entered the human race.

That night I was watching TV with my family. The dog was yapping at the door. Again. Yap yap yap. I'd had such a day. Jesus! Damn dog! Irritation welled up inside me. I took the remote control, pointed it at him, and pressed the mute button. Everyone laughed. Mommy was so silly. I went into the kitchen, cracked open a beer and wrote at the top of my shopping list "volcano ice blood ghost lion flames cave float love." Then I added "bananas, eggs, coffee." I would write a poem later.

I wandered around the kitchen, putting away dishes and wiping down the counters. What a day. It was *so* bad. Oh well, it was over. I leaned my elbows on the counter and added to my list "celery, Cheerios."

Doctors, the College, lawyers. Shit, the media. What a fucking circus. The headline in one paper this morning was "DOC STALKER." Why did they hate me so much? I should sue them too.

The phone rang. It was Jane, the woman who had encouraged me to get Blackwood out of my head by thinking about a tree. "Don't worry about the press, Sky. They don't matter. You know what's important. You know what the truth is. You know who loves you."

"Thanks Jane."

So none of it mattered. I knew I was loved. I could feel it. I shook my head in disbelief that such a wonderful thing could ever happen to me. What a gift.

Richard strode into the kitchen in his sweats and running shoes. "Off on my constitutional, honey."

"It's so dark out, wear that white sweatshirt, not the dark one, okay?"

"You mean the one that was navy blue but somehow got bleached in the wash and turned bright white? That one?" We laughed.

Jamie waltzed in and shouted "Hey Margie, Emma! Mommy and Daddy are having the laundry fight."

Richard and I looked at each other and smiled. Kids.

The house was finally quiet and I dragged my feet up to my study. I turned on the lamp and sat looking at the circle of light on the pad of paper on my desk. I caressed the page and felt its smooth white softness. At the top I wrote, "Above the Ice."

I never wanted to forget this day.

CHAPTER 31

BLACKWOOD'S DEFENCE HAD BEGUN. Judith told me not to go to the hearing so I sat at home in front of my computer trolling through the media coverage on the internet. "*Borderline Personality Disorder Patient Impossible to Treat*'" screamed out at me. The reporting was a brutal media circus, led by the ringleader Natty Hitchens. The victim, everyone guffawed, was a whacko. I was to blame, not the harmless Dr. Blackwood. Although I had been prepared from the outset for the label of Borderline Personality Disorder, nothing had prepared me for the contempt of the media. It felt like a medieval stoning. I knew women wouldn't ever report doctors, not now.

I drove through the gray city, clenching my jaw, as I dragged myself to lunch with Ann. Every now and then I let out a shaky sigh. I practiced my new mantra out loud: *I'm not nuts, what happened to me was nuts. I'm not nuts, what happened to me was nuts.* It was Ann who had taught me this, and it was true. It had been helpful. It still was. As I muttered, other drivers gripped their wheels and focused on the road. By the time I entered the darkened pub near High Park, my spirits were so low I could hardly move. My eyes probed through the blue haze of smoke and found Ann jumping in her seat, a big smile plastered on her face, barely containing her excitement. I inwardly rolled my eyes. Here we go. When I sat down, Ann leaned forward eagerly, her fingertips leaving greasy prints on the newspaper in front of her. She thrust it across the table, grinning away.

"Have you seen this? That article by Bicknell?"

"Oh yeah, I read it on the Internet. Horrible. All about how crazy I am."

The waitress came and took our orders. A western for Ann, Greek salad for me.

Ann saw I wasn't going to take the bait and shoved the newspaper right under my nose. The headline "Borderline Personality Disorder" stared at me. "The Internet doesn't show the pictures that go with the articles, does it?" Ann's mirth kept bubbling to the surface, erupting in little chirps.

It wasn't funny. The disorder, the reporter said, was impossible to treat and people who had it were manipulative. As if I could make Dr. Stubborn Blackwood do anything he didn't want to.

"No, they don't show the pictures. Why?"

"Open it up to the middle page spread." Ann was holding her breath so hard her eyes looked inflated.

I was already humiliated, why would I want to see more? Bloody Ann, stirring me up like this. I reluctantly obeyed. My eyes widened as looked at the two photographs. Unbelievable! I stared at the pictures and back at Ann. And then I tilted back my head and laughed and laughed.

Princess Di! Marilyn Munro! Borderlines! I roared until my stomach hurt. I couldn't believe the press. What idiots.

We propped the photographs against the ketchup. Every now and then one of us would dissolve into laughter, setting the other off. I put a piece of oregano from my Greek salad over my lip, puckered my mouth, and pretended I was Marilyn. Five minutes later Ann made a napkin crown and primped like Lady Di. We laughed our heads off.

And then suddenly it wasn't funny anymore. "Journalists have IQs of wombats," Ann snorted. "I mean, people with Borderline Personality Disorder can't maintain relationships. If a person can do this one thing, they don't have the disorder. They've seen your friends at the hearing. They know you've been married for decades. Like don't they get it?"

I tried to calm Ann down. "They're just trying to sensationalize their story."

But Ann was whipping up into a frenzy and ranted, "The *truth* is more sensational. That the College hires a psychiatrist who says their own witness is crazy? That the psychiatrists for both the defence and the College base the diagnosis not on assessing the victim, but on a chart written by an incompetent sexual abuser? That this is against the *Regulated Health Professions Act*? That there is systemic prejudice at the College against victims of sexual assault?" Ann was jabbing the air with her forefinger as she emphasized each point. "And why doesn't the lawyer for the College confine the testimony of the defence's psychiatrist to Blackwood's chart, where he wrote down everything he did to you? Where are Berka's fucking objections?"

The pounding waves of Ann's tantrum swept me up into her stormy tide. The system had let me down. The system had victimized me all over again. "Blackwood has the disorder, not me. He's Mr. Shout and Manipulate. On top of all that, the journalists know that neither psychiatrist has ever met me. Surely they know that giving a diagnosis is a restrictive act; the doctor has to have at least met the person before they can give a diagnosis. And then they can only give the diagnosis to the patient, not to a roomful of fucking strangers. Why doesn't the College follow the goddamn fucking law?"

"Yeah, yeah. And what did I say?" Ann lowered her voice to a deep conspiratorial whisper. "The College..." She gestured with her right hand, "The College..."

I joined in, "is not your friend."

Our hoots echoed around the pub. People were looking. We were much too loud.

"Oh Ann, why do people mock victims of sexual assault?"

Ann settled down and stirred her coffee. "People denigrate what they don't understand. They're frightened of the unimaginable, so to keep it away from them, to keep it from touching them, they blame the victim. And the more they're frightened of it, the more they denigrate and blame."

Made sense to me.

But then Ann revved up and began to rage again. "Well, it's pretty obvious Hitchens hates women and children. That's probably why she never married."

"Now Ann, we don't know the story of her life. Obviously something has gone very wrong for her."

"Naw, she's an asshole." Ann spit out the word with some pieces of egg. "Don't give me that compassion crap. Look what she's done to you. She deliberately and maliciously exposed enough details about you so there could be no doubt that you would be identified."

"Do you think she did it *on purpose*?" I was flabbergasted.

"Of course she did it *on purpose*," said Ann mimicking me. "Right after Blackwood gave his defence she wrote in her column something about wanting to scream your name from the treetops, or something like that. She wrote how unfair it was that his name wasn't protected by a ban. She's so stupid. She doesn't know all he had to do was ask for one. I think there's been a truly deliberate and malicious violation. Why don't you write to *Jerka* Berka and make a formal request that Hitchens' paper be charged with contempt of the publication ban?"

I agreed to do it. It sure would help other women in the future if reporters were more respectful of publication bans. "I guess that means I'm going to have to go through those awful articles and extract all the exposing details about me."

I was astonished that my publication ban had been *deliberately* violated. Who would *dare*?

I was talking to Marion on the phone.

"How are your kids getting through all this, Sky?"

"Well, actually, it's unbelievable, but they don't even know."

"What, they don't read the papers? It's pretty obvious it's you."

"That's why I'm calling. What do you think about me asking the College to charge Hitchens and the paper she works for with contempt of the publication ban?"

"Good idea," said Marion.

I said, "Well, I just think that many women go to their family doctors for therapy because they are in an abusive relationship with their husband, right?"

"Right."

"Right. Well, often these women have been abused as children and never learned about sexual boundaries. Like me. A doctor can merrily abuse away and the woman doesn't even know it's wrong."

Marion responded, "True. But then, if an abused woman eventually receives good help she may actually report the doctor to the College."

"Like me," I said. "The College assures her that her name will be kept private: the secret is safe. But many people think a doctor's abuse is a romantic sexual affair. If the abusive husband finds out about it from the press because of someone like Hitchens, he could well lose his temper, and not just beat his wife, but actually be so enraged as to *kill* her. By exposing personal, identifying details, Hitchens puts women at risk."

Marion said, "Stupid idiot."

"Hitchens wrote that publication bans are to protect children. So shallow. That's not nearly the whole story. Lives are at stake."

"Stupid fucking idiot."

I laughed right out loud. Marion *never* swore.

I dredged through Hitchens' prejudicial articles and made a long list of all the details she had revealed about me, causing me to be identified. Fuck her. I typed up a report and personally delivered it to Berka.

When Berka's responding email zapped into my computer, I saw that my sideline book, *Stupid Things Lawyers Say* was getting fleshed out. My mouth actually dropped.

Berka, a supposedly well-educated person, said that although I had been identified by the press during the first week of the hearing, she'd spoken to them, they'd apologized and now they were no longer violating the ban. Therefore they wouldn't be charged. I stared at the computer and just shook my head. The ban had *already* been violated. Pure and simple.

During the second week of Blackwood being on the stand, I decided, against Judith's advice, to show up for a few hours of his morning testimony. The papers had made me out to be so crazy that I dressed with care, putting on one of my new I-am-a-sane-person suits. And because Hitchens had commented on my shoes, I wore some new boots. I hoped they were cool. I was going to make an appearance.

I stood at the bottom of the stairs in my house and shouted up, "Bye kids. Daddy's making eggies. I'm off."

Emma called down, "Okay Mom, see you later."

Margaret asked, "Will you be home after school?"

"Of course honey, see you when you get home."

Jamie whined, "I don't like Daddy's eggies. He makes them too hard."

"But not scrambly eggies, sweetie. He's the best! Bye."

Richard came up and kissed me softly. "Good luck today. You know I don't agree with all this, but you're doing a good job."

"Thanks honey. Can you believe that after ten years of standing at the bottom of the stairs in my nightie and slippers, calling up "Eggies in one minute, breakfast," not one of our children has asked me where I am going?"

"Thank heaven for small miracles."

I sat, tucking my feet under my chair. Hitchens was standing by a doorway of the hearing room, talking to her sidekick, Bicknell, of the other national paper. These two journalists were damaging women more than they could ever dream. Between Bicknell's sensationalized Borderline Personality article and Hitchens' implication that the doctor was the victim, I felt nauseous. How could it possibly be that a trained professional, a doctor, was the victim of a vulnerable woman who had gone to him for a simple case of anxiety?

I could feel Bicknell's eyes on me and kept my head down. I unzipped my briefcase and took out two sheets of lined paper. Let him report that, I thought, let him report that the cuckoo lady can write. You betcha I can. Just wait and see. I'm going to write about how no one should ever believe the press, that "journalistic integrity" was an oxymoron. Ditch the "oxy" part, he was a moron.

Blackwood was on the stand wearing scuffed desert boots and the same rumpled blue suit. His faded cloth briefcase was slumped at his feet. Mr. Pathetic.

I listened in disbelief as he answered Keating's questions. No, he hadn't been sexually aroused, no he didn't look at me while I mastur-bated, no he hadn't touched my clitoris, no he didn't touch me on his own, I always guided his hand. Bleat after plaintive bleat, the baleful fellow was determined to look like the doctor who got in over his head and that the patient made him do it. I squirmed in my chair, making notes for Berka to use in her cross-examination.

During the morning break, Judy, Berka, and I were in a tiny board-room off to the right of the hearing room.

"I've made some notes about where he lied on the stand."

Berka looked up from her file and gave a condescending nod in my direction.

"He said I moved his hand down my back. What? Do I have rubber arms? Ask him about that, Berka. Ask him how I guided his hand to touch the back of my knee while I was lying face down on my front. That's in his notes. Him touching the back of my knee. It would be impossible for me to guide his hand there."

"I'll get him on other things. That would waste the College's time."

I sighed. Ann had warned me the College would say that, but I persevered. "He's a liar, Berka. Prove it."

She picked some lint off her suit.

I forged on, "And he didn't touch my clitoris? It's in his list! He wrote it down. Show him the list, Berka. Catch him in the lie."

Berka merely said, "I have my questions planned, don't worry."

But I was very worried. Berka's specialty was constitution law, for heaven's sake.

The next day I read Bicknell's headline: "*Accuser Takes Notes as Doctor Testifies.*" Ha ha, I was right. And apparently I had shaken my head dismissively. That was probably when Blackwood said he touched me with a "flat hand." He'd actually raised his hand and held it stiffly straight in front of the panel to show them what he meant. Nice try. It wasn't his hand that was stiff.

Natty Hitchens' reporting shocked me. Hitchens bought Blackwood's testimony, hook, line and sinker: he only wanted to help his patient; he felt he had to rescue me; he was so sorry he prolonged my suffering. My mind spun as I read in disbelief. How could he possibly think he was helping me by putting his fingertips on my nipples? Hitchens wrote that what happened was a function of my illness and his inexperience. And that in this, Blackwood was noble. *Noble?*

I felt like I'd been kicked in the chest. No one seemed to understand the impact of repeated, horrific, long-term sexual abuse on a psyche. I thought I was going to implode.

The next day my therapist friend, Catherine Thorne, called from Nova Scotia. "Boy oh boy, is that Hitchens ever a ball-licker."

I wondered what a "ball-licker" was and then started to cry, "She said he was *noble*."

"Don't worry about it. Hitchens is disturbed. There was a therapists' conference down here this weekend, and believe me, therapists across the country are disgusted by her reporting. They are writing in to the editor, don't worry. Therapists get it."

I decided to go down to the hearing again two days later. I listened incredulously as Blackwood testified that he had an erectile dysfunction. During a break I complained to Judith. "I can't believe it. He is such a liar."

Judith calmly reassured me, "Oh, they all say they can't get it up. If you ask me, that's why they have to abuse their patients. It's the only thing that works for them. Berka should ask him during her cross-examination if he sought medical attention for his condition. Maybe then it will come out he prescribed Viagra for himself. Big no no."

The days of Blackwood being on the stand stretched on and on, his pitiful eyes beseeching the panel. He insisted that he had provided good therapy to his patient and then openly wept with remorse for harming me. *What?* No one picked up on the incongruity.

CHAPTER 32

MONTH LATER THE cross-examination by Berka began. I waited anxiously for her to question him and, I hoped, expose him as a liar. He had said he hadn't touched my clitoris, but there it was in his notes. This was such an important point. On this alone he could lose his license. Would Berka expose him?

No.

During the cross examination, Berka did her best to get Blackwood to admit that he saw me after the therapy because he was trying to avoid me reporting him. I hadn't even thought of this. He was stringing me along so I'd eventually forget what had happened? Not bloody likely.

Blackwood disagreed, saying the dates were helpful to his patient. Then Berka tried to get him to admit he was sexually aroused by me and again he disagreed. Again he said he had an erectile dysfunction. Of course Berka didn't challenge him on this. After this Berka kept trying to show that he had encouraged me to masturbate for him. This was very important: if they weren't going to use the fact that he had touched my clitoris, in order to revoke his license, the College had to prove encouragement.

But then Hitchens judged me as if I were the one at fault. "The challenge with her was never to cheer her on, in anything, but rather to find a wall tough enough to slow her down."

When I read this, my heart sank. Hitchens hadn't been in his office. She hadn't heard how he had been the one to suggest that I have an orgasm in his office, that it would help me. That Blackwood and I had negotiated each and every sexual session. That we had talked about doing things in such a way so he wouldn't lose his license. That he kept saying it helped me because fantasy got me ready for the real thing. That he'd be with me in a very powerful way. That he made a nice little bed for me. He was more than encouraging. But then, did I ever say these things on the stand? Had Berka even asked me? I just didn't know; I had been pretty dissociated the whole time. It was such a drag to not be completely here.

I was so frustrated. Watching a patient masturbate time and time again was sexual abuse. The word "encourage" shouldn't even *be* in the legislation. It was only there in the spirit of protecting a doctor from a patient who flung off her clothes and started to masturbate, willy nilly, in front of him. How often did *that* happen? That didn't apply here, where there were numerous, orchestrated occasions. I decided I wouldn't go to the hearing anymore.

I hated the College.

Ann was drinking scotch and coffee. "Did you read Bicknell's article quoting Blackwood's receptionist, Lydia, that you were disruptive in the office?"

"Yeah, I did. No surprise that they didn't dig up anyone else to corroborate, I mean, if I were that disruptive, which I wasn't, they'd have lots of people to say I was crazy in the waiting room. I was there enough."

"Lydia lied because she wants to keep her job, that's all."

"Well, you said I'd be the only one telling the truth, and you were right. At least that black fog of guilt isn't going to settle on my mind for the rest of my life."

I wondered how Blackwood would live with himself, knowing he lied on the stand. But then, I thought, he's been a liar all his life. He spins lies like spiders spin webs. He spun me in his office and he spun me along on dates.

The spin doctor wouldn't even notice.

The next day Cindy Heffner, Blackwood's girlfriend, testified. After reading the newspapers I was once again appalled. Because of Cindy's testimony, the newspaper headline had switched from *Borderline Personality Disorder* to *Stalker*. I called Ann in despair. "I wasn't stalking him."

"Not at all. Stalking implies malicious intent. What you were doing might appear to be stalking, but no, you weren't stalking him. All victims do really weird things. But these things help the victim survive. I've just been reading something about victims who suffer from complex post traumatic stress disorder. They have something called a trauma bond."

"Trauma bond? What's that?"

"It happens after there's been repeated long-term sexual abuse on a psyche. Victims always behave in ways that make them lose their dignity. They are desperate to be safe so they do familiar things that will help them continue to feel worthless, which is safe and familiar. Plus, they all believe they love their abuser; to label it anything else is too frightening. Victims try to find out as much as they can about their perpetrator to keep this myth alive."

So all victims did odd stuff. I wasn't crazy. I wasn't *stalking*. I had a trauma bond.

"You know his girlfriend Cindy lied on the stand."

"What, you didn't leave balloons on his car like she said?" Ann laughed.

I remembered that night and grinned. "No, I did that. But I don't think she saw them like she said she did. I don't think she was at his house. Her car wasn't even there."

"So aren't you the little miss Trauma Bond Princess, driving all over town, recreating your worthlessness!" We laughed.

"Whatever. She also lied about the flower I sent him the next Valentine's Day, saying the two of them discovered it and threw it out. I know he came home alone and put the flower on his table, where it stayed for three weeks!" I remembered the wild visit, with Blackwood flapping his arms and stumbling backwards. Now I knew what he'd been frightened of; that I'd report him to the College.

Ann stubbed out her cigarette. "Did you tell Berka about all this? She can put you back on the stand as a rebuttal witness, you know."

"Yeah, I told her, and then she asked me how I knew he'd come home alone. I described watching him from across the park and saw him picking up the flower. She rolled her eyes..."

Ann laughed and then suddenly became angry. "Did you catch the reporting on Dr. Merriweather, the defence's poor excuse for an expert witness? That guy can be bought. Why does the College allow him to get away with saying the things he does? Talk about an abuse of power! Imagine comparing a patient with a Hollywood character? He does it every time. He did it to me, and now he's doing it to you. So predictable. What a jerk. He is so unethical. Imagine diagnosing someone you've never met with an incurable life long illness and then delivering that diagnosis to a roomful of strangers? That's against the RHPA on both counts. And it happens at a *hearing?*"

Ann was on a warpath. "And he bases his diagnosis on *Blackwood's* chart, a sexual abuser? I mean, let's get real here. Blackwood kept notes on how he sexually abused a woman. And *you're* crazy?"

Ann gulped down yet another spiked coffee and sucked on a cigarette so hard that the end glowed and sparked. But her tirade seemed to be over.

"I know, I know," I sighed. "I mentioned all this to Berka."

"So what did Berka the Jerka say?"

"She said, 'I won't even go there'!"

Ann's fury ramped up again. "She's ridiculous. Where the hell are her balls?" She slammed down her drink. "Merriweather is an asshole. Berka is an asshole. Keating is an asshole. Cindy is an asshole. The College is an asshole." Sparks and spittle flew.

I couldn't cope with Ann's rampant swearing and the room started to sway and tilt. I bleated, "The College needs a new reporting process."

Ann looked like she just might explode.

Finally the hearing was over. I was sickened by the whole process and reported Keating to the Law Society of Upper Canada for violating Rule Four of their Rules of Conduct. He had misled the panel by referring to me in almost every sentence he uttered as "the witness, who has a Borderline Personality Disorder..." when he knew there was no basis for that diagnosis. He was misrepresenting a witness, not allowed! And he knew that Dr. Merriweather was a charlatan, a purchased mouthpiece, who broke regulations governing his profession. That too was misrepresenting a witness.

The Law Society phoned me and said they had no jurisdiction over quasi-judicial settings. I was incredulous and asked them, "Even when a lawyer lies during a hearing?" The poor woman on the end of the line made choking embarrassed sounds.

I also reported both Keating and Berka to the Registrar of the College for not upholding the *Regulated Health Professionals Act*. They had allowed each of their expert witnesses, both medical doctors, to give a diagnosis of a person they had never met and then delivered that diagnosis to a roomful of strangers. I pointed out that this simply wasn't allowed under the *Act*. I even cited the section. There was no response.

Ann and I laughed uneasily over lunches as we waited for the panel's decision. Months went by. I knew it was going to be a tie. I felt I had the panel pegged. But Ann kept saying he would have to lose his license. "Zero tolerance," she would say, emphatically pointing her finger at me, "The College has *zero tolerance* for sexual abuse."

But I had observed that the process was deeply prejudiced against the victim. His license would be safe; I believed he'd just get a penalty of a year or something like that.

I wrote a submission to the College panel titled "Systemic Prejudice at the College Against Victims of Sexual Assault." No response. But surfing the net cheered me up. I Googled the newspapers' editorial pages and discovered I had many supporters who were livid that a vulnerable woman had been medicalized in the press. Some of the contributors said it shouldn't even be mentioned that I had a mental illness, if in fact I even did, because doctors should never be sexual with patients. Hitchens articles had stirred up a hornet's nest of hatred towards her. Therapists from all over the country wrote in saying she was way out of line in her column. So, the whole world wasn't crazy.

The deep core shaking that had started during January finally stopped in mid-April. Why were they taking so long?

I wanted to stop doing the homework Blackwood had assigned me where I was to correct in a fantasy how I had responded when he put his erection in my face. But when I was sexual with Richard, my homework still crept into my mind unbidden, and I wanted it to stop haunting me. I didn't want to fantasize being with disgusting Blackwood when I was with my lovely Richard. My trauma bond was made of steel.

And so I sat in front of Maggie and re-lived the event yet again while Maggie moved her fingers back and forth. After this therapy session the eight-year pattern of the tormenting sexual fantasy about Blackwood finally stopped gripping me. Bit by bit his impact on me was being dismantled.

I'd get better. I'd be able to be totally here. I knew it.

Finally the College's decision arrived. I carefully picked the envelope out of my rusting mailbox. The clang of the shutting lid didn't even register over my clanging heart. I opened the letter calmly, already knowing what it would say.

Guilty? What? *Guilty?* My heart soared! I started to cry.

Dr. David Blackwood was found guilty of sexual abuse *and incompetence!* I didn't even know they were going for incompetence. I joyfully read through the decision, quickly turning page after page. This was wonderful. I had won!

But then my world lurched to a stop. Attached to the end of the decision was a written dissent. Somehow the military guy and that corpulent fellow believed that Blackwood had not encouraged me to masturbate for him. It was just as I had predicted. What Neanderthals! In the dissent, they acknowledged that although Blackwood had negotiated the rituals with his victim, put a pillow on the floor for me, sat by my head, put his hand on my breast, and watched me over and over again, he hadn't encouraged me! *Really?*

The penalty? He couldn't practice for a year. His license wouldn't be revoked. A slap on the wrist. Just like he said.

"Hey Mom, what's this?" Margaret was standing at the kitchen counter where I had tossed the College decision. She was poking the envelope with her finger. "It looks important."

I tried not to snatch it away and kept a smile frozen on my face. "Oh, just the result of a case I was in. Against a doctor. For sexual assault. It upset me so I reported him."

Jamie and Emma had sauntered in to the kitchen, looking for an after school snack. Jamie was digging through the pantry, his back to me. "So, is that why you stopped your kids' column in the paper?" His mouth was now full of peanuts.

"Yeah." Less is more, I thought.

"Get lots of money?"

"That's not our business, Jamie," chastised Emma.

I laughed, "That's another case. A civil suit. This was a hearing by the people who are responsible for doctors and the way they behave."

"Let me know about the money one. I wanna go."

"We'll see," I said as the kids ambled out, hands clutching pieces of fruit.

So. Now they knew. A relief, in a way.

In the aftermath of the hearing, Ann and I debriefed over many toasted westerns. In August we split a dessert to celebrate my fifty-first birthday. But Ann remained furious and kept venting her wrath. *"Zero tolerance,"* she would say, banging on the table while I cringed.

It was so unjust. So wrong. Was there anything I could do? Ann kept up with all sorts of legal activities on the part of victims. "Ann, do you know anyone who is taking on the College for its prejudice and failure to follow the law?"

"It just so happens I do, this lawyer lady. I don't know too much about her case because she isn't allowed to talk about it, but I know she is trying to get a class action suit against the College together with victims who have gone through the process but have been met with prejudice. I know you're not happy with your verdict, but you should be. Most victims end up losing completely. Why don't you meet with her?"

"Do you think she'd talk to me?"

"Sure. Here's her number."

So I organized a meeting with the lawyer Ann suggested. She was an expert in College proceedings and was challenging them. Over our lunch she told me it was her opinion that the College decision was illegal. There was absolutely no basis in law for the finding. Of course Dr. Blackwood had encouraged me to masturbate and he should have lost his license. Unfortunately, she informed me, that because the defence had come forth with the penalty and the College had accepted it, there could be no appeal. That was the way the cookie crumbled in the land of the RHPA. The case could never be examined for illegalities. However, she explained, if the College hadn't accepted Blackwood's plea, then he would be able to appeal the College's decision, a process which could go on for years. Meanwhile, he'd be harming women. I was disgusted. Given that I nearly lost my life, he should have lost his license.

But then I asked her if Blackwood could be charged with new allegations. She smiled and said yes.

Hmmm.

That night, after the kids were sleeping and Richard was out on his walk, I thought about writing a new Letter of Complaint. As I sat at my desk I doodled a point or two. Blackwood had not been charged with touching my clitoris. This was a new allegation. There was solid proof. He'd written everything down. His license would be revoked. Women would be safe. But right now I was so tired of it all. I sighed. At least the College case was over and he'd be off the street for a year.

And now that the College case was finished, the civil suit could begin.

CHAPTER 33

I WAS SITTING AT my desk going through stacks of papers in my office for the civil suit. Pages and pages of lawyers' crap. Mediation brief this, discovery that, photocopies of everything. The verdict was in from the College and the lawyers for the civil suit were now going to face off. The one with the most paper would win.

Except I had the best paper. I had the verdict from the College. I waved it in the air triumphantly. Blackwood had been found guilty by his ruling body so the skirmish would be weighted in my favour. I imagined myself in a court of law. I dreaded the idea. More awful days on the stand. More awful days of looking at Blackwood's hands. More days of dressing up.

If I had to go, I would, but really I just wanted the whole thing to go away. I wanted a settlement.

And then I laughed. As if cash would compensate me for my losses. Whatever. I was so done with lawyers.

I went through their many monthly bills. Their fifty or sixty official statements of account. I owed them enough to buy a house. A cute little bungalow perhaps, in the suburbs. And just what had they done for me? After five years? And exactly what had they billed me for? I read over the items. Photocopying. Naturally. Emails. Phone calls. Filing. Reading my poems? *Really?* Meetings. Travel expenses. Couriers. Look at that! They'd billed me for a cheese tray!

Up until that second in time I thought my lawyers were the good guys. But I remembered that cheese tray. Jeff Duffy? He'd stuffed his face with gouda while he crossed his Calvin Klein socks, which, I remembered thinking at the time, cost more than my whole outfit. And while he was chewing a croissant, crumbs scattering everywhere, he was instructing me on how to be a witness. How to give just the facts.

He asked me, "Describe the anal rape scene."

I gulped, "We were trying to get me to deal with—'

"No, no, no," he interrupted, "Just describe it. Factually. He stood where, you stood where. He did what. You did what." He wiped his hands on a napkin.

"He stood right behind me. His body touched mine. His erection was pressed against my buttocks. I shut my eyes. He put his arm around my neck. He covered my mouth with his hand. I turned—-"

Duffy broke in, "You'll do. Cheddar? Or brie, perhaps."

I remembered that cheese tray, alright. Boy oh boy, did I ever. I also remembered that I, of course, had felt like throwing up and didn't touch a crumb. And they billed *me*?

I was sitting at a shiny mahogany table in a meeting room at the court house on Queen Street. My now grown-up son Jamie was waiting outside. He had driven me to this last ditch effort at a settlement before we all trekked off to court. I was too nervous to drive because Blackwood would be there. Lawyers and paper surrounded me while at the head of the table sat a retired judge. Blackwood was in the same rumpled suit. There seemed to be some kind of verbal arm wrestle going on between the lawyers. They were negotiating a settlement amount. Sums of money were tossed out, pencils scratched at pads of paper, and heads shook dismissively. Finally a puny offer was made by Blackwood's lawyers.

I nearly laughed.

The judge perhaps sensed my mood and said, "You should accept this, given your behaviour."

Blackwood looked at me smugly.

Duffy said, "We will adjourn for a few minutes to consider this."

No, I thought, we'll adjourn so I shriek in private! With red hot anger zinging through my body, I strode into the hall and spat out the pathetic amount to Jamie.

"Your lawyers have done a terrible job. Blackwood harmed you way worse than this. You couldn't work. This case should have been settled years ago. The amount is ridiculous. Ask for more." He was adamant.

I'd calmed down. What a great kid. "It's so nice that you are protective of me Jamie, but you know, I did some pretty crazy things."

But Jamie was clear, "Yeah, that was Blackwood's fault. Ask for more."

I fiddled with my wedding ring, turning it over and over. Should I?
Then the cheese tray soared across my mind like a random frisbee. I
had suffered enough. Yeah, I'd ask for more.

"Okay."

And I got a little more. After the paltry check arrived in the mail I
paid off a quarter of the huge line of credit that we'd started when I
stopped working.

It didn't matter. It was over.

Marion and I were having lunch at her place. She listened carefully as
I rattled on and on. Everything was over.

"I'm sorry I'm talking so much Marion."

"It's okay Sky, it's good to talk."

"Ten years have gone by since that first day I entered Blackwood's
office, unwrinkled and lithe, just turned forty-one years old. In six
months I'll be fifty-two. I've lost ten years of my life. My children
grew up while I drove around Blackwood's house, shouting conversations with him. While I played The Blue Car Game. While I
felt as if my skin was burning off my bones and I walked through
fire. While I couldn't touch or be touched. While I drank and wept,
whispered and wrote. Every night I scratched out shitty poems.
Weeping and whispering and writing. I almost killed myself because
of that man.

Marion said, "I know, but it's all over. And look what you have
accomplished! Despite everything, you have three great kids. And
maybe you'll write a book. It would help all kinds of people.
Women."

"Well, I sure hope so, otherwise there'd be no point. What doctors
do behind shut doors has to be stopped. Thanks for listening, as usual.
You're a good friend."

"So are you, Sky, so are you."

Marion had finished her whole sandwich and I hadn't taken a bite,
I'd been so busy gabbing away.

But now I knew what I had to do. One out of two women in therapy
were abused by their doctor. Some of them died. I would write a book
about how I was doctored. About the impact. About the prejudice.
About how often it happens to women.

Maybe it would change a few things. Maybe it would help women.

I sat in front of my computer and typed "Chapter One" and was immediately seized by panic. What if I couldn't do it? I was *stupid stupid stupid*. I'd let a doctor run his hands all over my body. I fell in love with an abuser. How stupid could you get?

Sky, get a grip! You're not stupid. You kept going back because you didn't know it was abuse. You had no way to know. You were used to it. It was comforting. Plus you were kind and felt sorry for him. And falling in love? You had to believe you were in love with him because it masked your terror. You were spellbound by a trauma bond. *Get a grip. Move ON.*

And then my fingers flew over the keyboard. The book fell out of me as if it were already written. The words appeared one after another in rapid fire succession on my computer screen. I didn't refer to a single file, not one. I knew what had happened to me. Oh boy, did I know.

That night Richard poked his head into my office and asked me over the noise of the tapping keys, "What are you writing?"

"Nothing much."

"You're working on that book, aren't you?"

"What book?' I turned around to look at him, my back blocking the screen so he couldn't read Blackwood's name. "How was your day, sweetie?"

"How's the book going?" Marion looked at me carefully, her eyes searching deep into mine, looking for signs of distress. "You've been working on it for months."

I could feel my face crumpling as I spoke. Writing it was so hard. "Oh, Marion, I was writing the awful bit about me rocking back and forth in my office, whispering in the dark, 'Who is the man? Who is the man?'"

Marion sat very still, her hands on the table, waiting for me to continue.

"Well, when I write it all out, I can see the sequence of events. I started whispering 'who is the man' and rocking back and forth right after Blackwood rewired me. Blackwood told me the man was my father. It wasn't, I know that now. Today it hit me that the man was *Blackwood! He* was the one abusing me. *He* was the one standing behind me, pressing his erection into my bum as he rewired me. Fear is licking my arms as I say this." I rubbed my arms and Marion leaned over and rubbed them too.

"You got away, Sky. He can't hurt you now. You're okay. I always knew he was the man, but I didn't want to tell you. I was worried it would frighten you."

"I'm so angry he said 'the man' was my father. My poor Dad. Blackwood damaged my whole family."

Marion sat up straight and cleared her throat. I looked at her questioningly, "What?"

"Well," said Marion, "We-l-l, I was wondering if you've figured out who was abusing you in your bed when you were little?"

"Oh. It was..." I looked off into the distance as I reached deep into my mind. I saw myself sleeping in that far-off bedroom at the age of eleven. I heard the stairs creak and felt TV snow tugging at a corner of my skull. Who? Who had taken off my underwear and thrown it on the floor?

Marion watched me carefully, knowing I was delving into an awful, dark past.

I suddenly thrust my fist into the air and shouted victoriously, "Lynny-poo! It was Lynny-poo!"

One afternoon I was feeling low. I had been working on the section in the book about the College's ridiculous decision and called Marion to give myself a boost.

She soothed me. "You didn't lose your case, Sky. Blackwood *was* found guilty of sexual abuse *and* incompetence."

"I know, but it's atrocious that I was made out to be the crazy lady that made him do it. He should be in jail."

"There's no statute of limitations for sexual assault, Sky. You can go to the police anytime. He would be found guilty."

"I know, I know. But right now I'm not going to make a career out of what Blackwood did to me. He has already stolen ten years of my life."

"Why don't you look at his penalty again."

"What? To cheer myself up?" I laughed. "Most people would go out for a drink."

That night I did both: I had a drink while I read *all* the penalties of *all* the doctors over the last two years. It took me a couple of hours to fish through the College web site. Only one doctor had a penalty more severe than Blackwood's!

That cheered me up. Sort of.

The summer was coming and the book wasn't finished. I needed a quiet place to focus. So I packed up my car and drove out to my cabin by the sea. I didn't have any kids with me this time. Somewhere along the way they'd grown up and were now working at summer jobs. I set up my ten-year-old laptop on a wobbly plywood table by the woodbox and found an old paint-splattered chair to sit on. Heaven. While I worked I could hear the ocean breathing on the cobblestone beach down the hill. The sounds of the watery landscape enveloped me and permeated my soul with soft beauty. An emptiness that had been in me was filling up with the holy spirit of the universe while I sat in my little shack by the sea, making sense of what had happened to me.

Every day for the next three weeks I woke up, went for a run, and then sat at my computer until noon. I took an afternoon break, ate dinner, walked to the wharf to watch the sunset, and then was back at it. I pushed my fingers to move quickly over the keyboard; I wasn't going home until I was done and I'd promised my family I'd be back before my birthday in August. I often worked late into the night and could hear the lobster fishermen on the wharf loading up their boats, getting ready to head out into the dark.

Finally it was finished. Hooray!

I celebrated by going to the beach. I grabbed my lunch, knapsack, and beach chair and walked down the path through the mossy woods to the sea, sandals squelching in the muddy track. I lugged my stuff across an iron-red stream, my feet sure and strong on the rocky bed. Finally I was where I wanted to be, where the sand stretched for miles all around me, white and firm. Where the sky was huge and I was humbled by the magnificence of the land. Where I was now free from Blackwood being in my head and the land and the spirit of nature was back, right where it belonged. The ocean breeze flapped my long sleeves as I set up my chair. I stuffed one end of my umbrella into a lobster trap so the wind wouldn't blow it over, sat down, covered my legs with a towel, pulled my hat low over my forehead, put on my sunglasses, and reached into my knapsack for my turkey sandwich, salad, and trashy mystery novel. Perfect. Richard would have hooted at my getup. I was going to enjoy the sun!

I gazed at the clear blue line of the ocean's horizon. That's where I write, I thought. I turned my head from left to right and saw that it was an arc. It was reaching its arms around me in an embrace. Funny how I had never noticed that before. The horizon wasn't a straight line, it was a curve.

I would soon be fifty-two. I had almost lost my life, my husband, my children. I temporarily lost my religion and my mind. My career was in ruins. Over ten years of my life, gone. I asked myself if I was angry. Well, maybe a little. I was sad, yes. Philosophical, maybe some days. But I knew in the marrow of my bones that it wasn't my fault.

As I sat on the beach chewing my delicious sandwich and eating my salad, I asked myself how I *really* felt, in this moment, right now.

I smiled to myself, shaking my head in disbelief. "I am so *lucky*. So, so lucky I didn't die. Unbelievable!" I stretched my feet out in front of me into the sand. "My husband loves me and I love him. My kids are fine. God is in nature. I can write."

My eyes rested on the blue line of the horizon that wrapped around me. I knew how I felt. I was really, really grateful to finally be *here*.

ACKNOWLEDGEMENTS

A heartfelt thanks to my loyal friends who stood by me for years while I was suffering from Post Traumatic Stress Disorder. I don't know what I would have done without you. A special thanks to Kerry Tobin, who supported me daily and is a truly generous soul.

Many people helped shape this book. I am indebted to my sensitive and talented editors at Inanna Publications. I would also like to thank Pamela Tate and Sue Garratt Elsey for the hours and hours they spent editing the various stages of the manuscript. Their insight and grace were very appreciated. Susan Marcus, Peggy Hutchison, Barbara Burt, Barb Symmons, and John Dunworth all gave valuable comments on early manuscripts which I appreciated. Thanks to Elizabeth McKenna. I hope this book helps women as much as she helped me.

I would also like to thank the investigator and the victim support person at the College of Physicians and Surgeons of Ontario for always treating me with compassion, respect, and dignity.

And last but not least, I am very grateful to Inanna Publications for publishing a book such as this. Thank you.

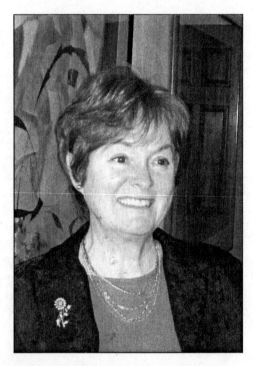

Sky Curtis is a former magazine writer, educational software designer, editor, playwright, columnist and children's writer. She now writes fiction and non-fiction books for adults. She lives in Toronto with her family.